WHERE MYSTERY DWELLS

B. J. F. LAUBSCHER

WHERE MYSTERY DWELLS

A Psychiatrist studies Psychical Phenomena

Preface by
Canon John D. Pearce-Higgins

JAMES CLARKE & CO., LTD.
CAMBRIDGE & LONDON

This Edition 1972

SBN 227 67801 X

Printed in Great Britain by
Redwood Press Limited
Trowbridge, Wiltshire

CONTENTS

INTRODUCTION

The reader will find that this book has emerged from that particular cradle of experience, which modern society has swept from the highways of true knowledge. The evidence contained in its pages will I hope contribute towards the birth of a new attitude of mind among those who value thought and its influence on man's consciousness.

It is my hope that the work of the forgotten psychic research pioneers will be consulted, since the factual evidence of their discoveries should serve as the starting points for new discoveries and research.

There is no reason why the principles of science impartial and progressive in the search of new truths, free from prejudice, should not be consistently and sympathetically applied to research in psychic phenomena.

In psychiatry, psychology, Biology and Philosophy we should not pretend to be able to interpret the nature of man, while we exclude supernormal psychic phenomena from the sources of our knowledge.

The evidence which moved me to put my thoughts in writing is concerned with the innate reality of the self. There are in every walk of life increasing numbers of people who cannot think of their total annihilation at death. These questioning minds as well as the occurrence of various psychic phenomena from poltergeists to ectoplasmic forms which vanish into thin air are surely worthy subjects for research.

It would be welcomed if the opening of these channels of thought could lead to departments for psychic Research at our universities. I would especially prefer to see research in ectoplasmic manifestations, clairvoyance and astral projections. Mediumistic persons capable of such manifestations should be employed, encouraged and adequately remunerated by such departments for psychic research.

For this purpose it would be necessary to establish a fund and entrust its management and the control of the work to the "South African Society for Psychic Research". I believe such research will provide new evidence on which we can build a better understanding of man's real nature and perhaps in the end produce evidence for an "Advanced Science of Psychobiology". Such a science will enlarge our comprehension of the self and assist in the promotion of a higher humanity.

It will certainly assist, judging by the evidence I have found, to counterbalance our lopsided aggressive impulses by means of spiritual factors having the approval if not the authority of science.

The hundreds of people who have written to me have shown how many of them feel the need for a different approach to these unfamiliar happenings so that correct interpretation can add to our knowledge.

I am indebted to all my correspondents who so kindly wrote to me of their experiences. I am especially grateful to the press for placing my need for certain information before the public. But as always there are certain individuals whose assistance one must value in a special manner. In this regard I have pleasure in thanking Mr. M. M. Sadie, 39 Keston Crescent, Marlborough, Durban, for his most informative Afrikaans manuscript dealing with his psychic investigations. He placed this at my disposal to select from it what I required. Mr Sadie had collected some remarkable cases.

Mr. N. L. Mansvelt, Box 69, Piet Retief, who so kindly loaned me books from his private library and last but not least my sincere thanks to Mrs. G. G. Jenvey who typed my manuscript as her contribution towards an enhancement of man's world of knowledge.

B. J. F. LAUBSCHER

PREFACE

I feel very honoured at being asked to write the preface for the English edition of Dr. B. J. F. Laubscher's book, which was first published in 1963 in South Africa. Dr. Laubscher is a leading psychiatrist, a former president of the South African Red Cross, and also a student of comparative anthropology, whose first book was about the Xosa culture, and he is a doctor of distinction. His qualifications and standing are of importance when it comes to assessing the value of a work of Parapsychology, not least since he is a qualified medical psychiatrist entering upon a field which is little considered by his colleagues. While a goodly number of eminent scientists have in the past embarked upon the study of psychic phenomena with a view to the debunking of them, and yet having 'come to scoff have remained to pray', Dr. Laubscher is unusual in that having been brought up among the native people on a South African farm, he has been familiar with the phenomena since childhood, and therefore does not appear to have that built-in resistance to the subject which is commonly found among European and American researchers.

One of the most interesting features of the book is the amount of refreshingly unfamiliar material taken from his experiences in South Africa, many being from his own clinical practice. There are examples from personal experience of almost every type of psychical phenomena, but if one were to single out the main theme of the book it is the concern for the reality and significance of the 'astral' or 'etheric' body, as evidential for survival, both from out of the body cases, and also from the study of materialisations and apparitions. It is significant also that a doctor, concerned with the healing of the body, should plead for medical science to consider very seriously the possibility of 'ectoplasm' as a component or integral factor in the healing processes, whether spontaneously evoked or after injury or operation. Chapter X which deals with this point is written entirely from the medical standpoint by one who is fully familiar with the latest scientific studies, and when such a writer pleads for the serious consideration of the possibility of discovering new energy patterns such as the presence of ectoplasm and the etheric body would appear to imply, his arguments surely deserve the attention of his colleagues. The recent successful experiments in England of Mr. Colin Brookes Smith, working on the basis of K. J. Batcheldor's psychological insights, in producing physical phenomena under control conditions, would appear to give corroborative support to Dr. Laubscher's tentative hypothesis.

A preface should not be a review, yet it is difficult to avoid saying that I do not think I have ever read a more readable or fascinating study on this whole subject, and I can only hope that medical and psychiatric colleagues will give this book the attention which it deserves.

Theologians will also find much new grist to their mill. I am delighted that as a Christian layman Dr. Laubscher, both in this book, and in his other books, *Beyond Life's Curtain* and *In Quest of the Unseen*, crosses swords with current theological views and criticises them for their failure to consider or deal with psychic phenomena as facts in natural theology when presented in such a way as they are in this book or in other reputable psychic writings.

Clearly it will take much time to break down the inspissated prejudices and preconceptions of centuries of theological speculation, and since so much of the barrage of psychic literature makes little impact because of its unscientific and inadequate presentation of the material, the more books of the quality of *Where Mystery Dwells* that are made available, the better.

Continual dropping wears away the stone—no doubt the Church needed to be founded on the Petrine stone or rock—but unless this rock changes its shape very considerably under the impact of modern scientific knowledge, instead of being a refuge and a shelter, it may end by being a stone of offence, and indeed an obstacle to religious belief in a world of ever-changing and expanding human consciousness.

JOHN D. PEARCE-HIGGINS

Southwark Cathedral S.E.1.
May 1971

CHAPTER I

THE BEGINNING OF A SEARCH

I spent the early years of my life on a farm facing that tongue of the Atlantic ocean which with its tip at the mouth of the Berg River, formed St. Helena Bay.

The far distant horizon was ever a line of vision and, with its blue mountains gave a frame to the picture of the Bay.

Along the shore lived the coloured fisherfolk in their stone cottages, and there were also white fishermen and sturdy Italians and Sicilians. I learned to fish and sail with them in their long boats.

And when the wind blew squalls across the Bay we would tack hither and thither and then suddenly, with flapping sails and dipping oars, we would shoot into calm waters through a narrow rocky entrance. The seamanship and skill of these coloured fishermen always filled me with admiration. I enjoyed being with them. They provided adventure and their stories were often hair-raising.

These people lived on our land on a feudal system. They paid no rent and had free firewood and water but, during the harvest time they had to provide labour; besides this they paid a tithe of a tenth of the fish caught.

In those days I remember seeing up to twenty men marching forward, swinging their scythes and mowing down the golden wheat, while others followed, made and bound the sheaves with bands of straw. Others bent low would work with the sickle and so in a hive of industrious exertion and sweat, there was humour, good food and wine before the huge orange sun dipped behind Koringberg. Then when the harvest was in came the harvest feast. This feast itself was a tradition kept by my family. Whether they had brought this custom from Germany about three hundred years before, I do not know.

But when the harvest was in and the sheaves were stacked, then the coloured folk gathered, meat was roasted and wine was drunk. A sweetish red wine which they loved so much. The guitars concertinas and drums bewitched a people whose life was rhythm and song. The dance was on, all were gay. But the moment there was a fight my father administered justice, and the culprits were locked in the wagon-house until they repented.

My father was "Seur" and his sons were the "Klein Seurs." The Afrikaans tradition demanded sometimes painfully, that all addressed every coloured man who was our senior in years as

Outa, and every coloured female of the same status as Aia. I at least, was always conscious that these terms meant my respect for the dignity of the person.

One could never be rude or cross with a person whom you addressed either as Outa or Aia. I believe the ancient Hottentots called an elderly person Ta, and Outa hence signified a person who should be addressed and treated with respect.

Out of all these memories of what is now a bygone age, I retain many vivid impressions. One in particular has an emotional atmosphere of spirituality which even as a child, made me think that somewhere, transcendent to all earthly pleasures was a world where beauty, grace, and harmony ruled supreme and this I must add, was not taken from any religious teaching or traditional Biblical presentation.

I remember waking up one Christmas eve fairly far into the night, when I heard the strumming of guitars and melodious voices in sweet harmony. It took me a few moments to find my relationship to wakefulness. I thought of some enchanted dream. My bedroom was near that of my parents'. I went to the window and there in the moonlight, stood a large number of coloured men and women : fisherfolk and farm workers with sobbing concertinas and subdued, humming guitars; with voices blended by instinct and feeling, swelling into emotional power that was virtually palpable. They came to my father's bedroom window, late at night to sing "Silent Night, Holy Night." And then they disappeared quietly into the darkness. The next morning there were the greetings and our material appreciation.

The coloured people had a phantasy world which was almost a second world for dramatisation of deeds and fulfilment of dreams and desires. This world, therefore contained all the daring exploits and feats of courage with which the person longed to impress his fellowmen.

Strangely enough even as a boy, I knew this intuitively. We were so much together that I often identified myself with their animated imaginations; but then there were also the stories of phantoms seen of the dead who came back and wandered about the stables; and others from the next world who were malign and predatory.

But there were occasions when the voices were hushed in my presence and I sensed some secret which I was not to know. My insistence ultimately persuaded Outa Jantjes, who was my favourite to impart the secret on payment of a piece of ropey strong vile-smelling Boer tobacco. I then learned that they did not want to frighten me but one of the new men had seen the woman and child again early that morning.

I had of course heard about these phantom beings, because from time to time, some servant or other would speak about seeing a woman clad only in a short skirt, with a child held by the hand, running and disappearing into the side of the hill. No one took this seriously but this new servant was really very frightened and was telling the story when I arrived and the voices were hushed.

Now Outa Jantjes came of a family who, according to tradition, had been with my ancestors since their liberation as slaves. He always claimed to be a pure-bred Hottentot. I do not know if he was, but there was something distinctive about him. His cheek bones were prominent but his eyes were clear and not screwed up with wrinkles like those of Bushman blood.

His face too was longer and his chin broader, while his skin was a light brown; his body more muscular and his height greater than any Bushman's I knew. He boasted that he had no blood from the "Dies Volk", meaning the white race, and when he used the exclamation—"Hotnot"—one knew it was something that has been done par excellence; an outstanding achievement indeed. This then implied that only the real pure Hottentot could do such a thing. He had no equals.

I remember at a tender age being given many pickabacks by Outa Jantjes when I would twirl my fingers through his peppercorn hair. He was good-natured and his stories of talking animals could go on and on for hours as I sat and listened to him while he was leisurely mending harnesses.

Then came a day when a new stable had to be built for we were also breeding mules, and this was the time when the brown mule-teams of the Malmesbury district were the pride of the Western Province. The new stable was for a fresh mule-team to pull the huge wagon loaded with barrels of wine from Malmesbury to St. Helena Bay. Outa Jantjes loved those trips and would tell the most extraordinary stories of happenings along the road—embellishments which often amused my father.

Anyway, we were making bricks for the new stable and dug a deep hole into the very hillside where the traditional phantoms of running woman and child always disappeared. Outa Jantjes was in charge of the brickmaking and the filling of the moulds with clay while I sat nearby listening to the stories. Because on such occasions when they were working in a group and close together the fountain of stories never ran dry. I had by this time accepted the world of ghosts as some sort of reality.

Sitting there and absorbed in their doings I suddenly heard a shout from the hole in the hillside. They had come upon something startling. I went forward and there we saw a collection of bones and two skulls deep down in an ant bear hole. This was about twelve feet from the surface and meant that the front part of the hole must have collapsed many years before.

Outa Jantjes would not let them touch the bones until the Seur had given instructions. My father was called. The examination showed a skeleton of a person of small stature and one other of a very small person undoubtedly a child. The bones were all disjointed but strangely some of the ribs were still in place whereas the skulls too were well preserved.

My father ordered Outa Jantjes to collect the bones in a bag and to make a box and bury the remains in the burial-place reserved for the coloured people. I assisted Outa Jantjes in the making of the box and we even attempted to make it look like a coffin. We placed some straw in the box and laid the bones neatly on the straw with the two skulls close together. That afternoon he dug the grave and we carried the box with its skeletons to the burial-ground.

There Outa Jantjes insisted that I should say a prayer as this was always the duty of the Seur or his sons. But I did not know what to say so Outa Jantjes told me to ask the Lord to tell the owners of the skeletons that we had given them a better burial than they would have had from their own people, and that they must go and rest and not keep running towards the hill and frightening people; also that I must not forget to say Amen for that would mean that we have done a good job and that the Lord approves.

I managed to tell the Lord all these things and if I hesitated Outa Jantjes prompted me in whispers. It seemed to me quite awesome as if the Lord was kindly listening to Outa Jantjes and me, and was satisfied.

But as we walked home Outa Jantjes winked at me and patted the leather pouch which he wore on his belt. He swore me to secrecy and produced two little finger bones. He had kept these because he wanted to find out who they belonged to and how they had got into an ant bear hole. He would tell me later how this information was to be obtained, but it might be as well for me to be at the cellar that evening when the wine and food rations were being given out after the day's work.

The others drank out of cups but Outa Jantjes had a horn which hung on the wall and he only drank out of the horn. Now his ration was the horn half-full but when I drew the wine for him I always filled the horn when no one was looking. My delinquencies were largely concerned with obtaining extra wine and tobacco for Outa Jantjes. My reward was a fount of stories.

I do not remember how long after this event it was when Outa Jantjes told me that the man who could decipher the history of the skeletons would visit his house. But I would have to provide at least half a bottle of wine and a fairly large piece of Boer tobacco. It took me several days to collect the wine which usually dripped from the tap into a receptacle, to obtain almost a full bottle. The tobacco was also obtained by surreptitious means.

Then one Saturday afternoon Outa Jantjes quietly told me to bring the wine and tobacco to his house in the valley that evening when all had retired to bed. As my room opened onto the stoep I tiptoed out into the dark for Outa Jantjes' little mud house.

There was a most disquieting feeling in the air and I imagined myself as being accompanied by the spirits who owned the skeletons. Every bush portrayed a sinister figure, and then to crown it all the "news carrier" bird, which flies by night and wails a most forlorn cry, telling of someone about to die just then flew overhead. I felt that every omen was against me. I was deeply steeped in the second world of Outa Jantjes.

At last I reached his house and found a queer wizened-looking Bushman with a face wrapped in wrinkles which made his watery eyes mere slits, sitting on his haunches while before him were lying several small knuckle bones of animals. He was talking about the ailments of one of the women, and then he gave her some roots and herbs out of his leather bag to cook and drink.

I handed Outa Jantjes the wine and the tobacco. He first took a long swig at the bottle while the bone-thrower's eyes stared at him. Then the bone-thrower stretched out his hand and deftly dislodged with a sucking sound the bottle from Outa Jantjes' mouth. He put almost the whole neck of the bottle into his mouth and just allowed the wine to run down his gullet.

Then he filled his clay pipe with the tobacco which I had brought, and as he smoked the dense fumes of the tobacco were blown through his nostrils, reminding me of the picture of a dragon snorting fire, which I had seen on someone's dressing-gown. Outa Jantjes said that I must not be in a hurry because the Bushman could only think properly when his brain was full of smoke.

He sat and puffed for what seemed an age; then he held out his hand and Outa Jantjes placed the two little finger bones therein. He never opened his eyes. In any case, one never knew when they were open for even when he was looking the lids were still lying almost on top of each other. He just sat blowing volumes of smoke out of his broad flat nostrils while occasionally without opening his mouth he spat through his front teeth a long stream of yellow-brown tobacco juice right into the fire about ten feet away.

It made a "shreet" sound and as the spittle reached the red coals it sizzled. I was quite fascinated by the accuracy of this man—spitting with apparently closed eyes without looking up straight into a small fire in the fireplace.

Then holding the little finger bones in his closed hand he began to talk in his quaint Afrikaans. The bones "told" him of something which had happened many many years ago—long long before the white man had come to that part of the country. The bones said there was a tribe of Hottentots living very comfortably near the Berg River mouth. Their captain was a clever man and he followed in his father's footsteps by remaining near the river and making that land with its great "vleis" their preserve.

They made their huts of laths cut from long green sticks, and then after bending them and tying their tops in the framework of a hut, they covered them with grass-woven mats. Their women were very good at weaving these mats.

They trained their cattle and tamed them so that they responded to the various whistling commands of the Hottentots. The cattle participated in their warfare since the Hottentots always attacked from the protection of their charging cattle, and these were controlled and directed by the different whistled commands. They took great pains to train the cattle and their oxen were almost pets since all their belongings—mats, clay pots and calabash utensils as well as the lath-like sticks for making the huts were packed on the backs of their oxen whenever they moved camp—for it was the custom not to remain in one place too long even if they moved only a short distance away.

There were always enemies and if they moved frequently they were alert and were not taken by surprise. These people only fought when their preserves were invaded. They put up certain signs for their boundaries—perhaps two branches tied together. That was what he "saw" from the bones of the skeletons.

These Hottentots like the Bushmen also used long bows and arrows, and they also poisoned the tips just like the Bushmen. He saw a picture of some Bushmen finding an ox belonging to the Hottentots. They killed this ox and had a feast. The Hottentots went on the spoor and came upon the place where the ox had been eaten. They immediately prepared for war to exterminate the Bushmen who had invaded their preserves.

They found the Bushmen tribe who were fighting a rear-guard action in order to allow the women and children to escape into the kloofs of Koringberg. But the charging cattle of the Hottentots were close on their heels coming on in a half-moon with their long horns well down. The Hottentots were shooting showers of arrows over their heads at the retreating Bushmen who were not only more fleet of foot but far more dexterous with bow and arrow on the run than their pursuers.

At last as they gained the high ground where our farm now stood the Hottentots were upon them and several Bushmen were shot, wounded and trampled to death by the charging oxen. A woman and her child lagged behind from exhaustion, and as the charging cattle came near they dived into an ant bear hole in the side of the hill but unfortunately for them they were seen. The Hottentots closed the mouth of the hole with stones and stamped on it for the earth to collapse and so the Bushman mother and child died of suffocation. The fear of that moment made them repeat the scene of their death for many many years.

All this was beyond my comprehension for how could a man obtain all that information by merely holding the finger bones in his hand? All that the bone-thrower would say was that the bones "told" him. But Outa Jantjes said it need not be bones it could be anything because the Bushman could feel what had happened to things and who were associated with the object.

I had a clasp-knife with a mother-of-pearl type of handle given to me by an uncle who fought in the Anglo-Boer war and who had been badly wounded. His one leg was shorter than the other and he walked with a limp. I handed the bone-thrower my knife. He did not even examine it; he merely held it in his hand while he blew smoke through his nostrils and occasionally "shreet"-spat across the room into the fire on the other side. He said the knife was a present from a man who had fought in the war and who was big and heavily built. He had been shot through the thigh and had fallen from his horse. The English had picked him up and sent him to their hospital and he drew a cross on the floor and said it was red. He gave me back my knife and said that I would lose it before long which I did.

That night I lay awake until I heard the cocks crowing. How did this man know? How could he tell all these things by merely touching an object; since his story about the knife was correct in every detail why should his story about the Bushman skeletons not be true? But how did he do it? What made him different from me and gave him powers of mind which I had not?

Surely this story could not be in the knife nor the other in the finger bones? When I told my family about the bones they said it could not be verified and that they had not heard about Hottentots having trained their cattle to charge in formation and respond to whistling commands. Well years later I spoke to an archivist who told me that there were records of Huguenot observations that the Hottentots actually did do all these things as told to me by the bone-thrower : a few hundred years later this illiterate Bushman spoke about knowledge which we did not possess. There was also no traditional need why he should have remembered ancient Hottentot customs.

Naturally I imagined some magical way of knowing these

matters. Outa Jantjes had told me that these people knew the art of magic and how to employ it. Somehow at the back of my mind remained this unfathomable world of impressions in a knife and the bony remains of Bushmen. Did the story of these running phantoms which disappeared into the hill perhaps give the Bushman a clue? But there was something else which the Bushman had told us. He said that he could visit places in his dreams, and he could meet people from far away in his dreams and talk to them. He could even talk to the spirits of the dead in his dreams.

All these things were not only puzzling but I had no way of understanding them and when I spoke to people about them they kindly pointed out that "that way lies madness." This made me think that there was this strange world of invisible beings and doings but that one must avoid this at all costs. I went away to school and had less opportunity to share certain thoughts with Outa Jantjes, and others of his class.

Then one day during school holidays Outa Jantjes told me that the bone-thrower was coming to see him after attending to a coloured girl named Grietje who was possessed by an evil spirit. I had forgotten about the bone-thrower; at least when in the end I could not understand how these powers came about I began to wonder whether one should bother; they seemed so impossible, perhaps they were not true at all. Who knows Outa Jantjes and the bone-thrower could have concocted the whole thing just to obtain wine and tobacco! But once I had been reminded of his visit my doubts came back and my mind was not so keen to explain away the strange happenings and the description of my uncle and his wound.

I learned that Grietje was the daughter of a fisherman. At least he had married her mother when she was a little girl. Actually the story was that Grietje was illegitimate and the child of a Sicilian fisherman. I went to their house on my way to do some rock fishing. I found Grietje an attractive coloured girl of the near-white group. She had long eyelashes which were of a fluttering nature and she was very shy. She looked slyly at one and more often down than up. Her hair was smooth, long and pitch black. She was sturdily built but I could not miss the impression of coyness or mischief which her personality conveyed although she hardly spoke a word.

I was told by her mother that for no reason at all stones were thrown on the roof, and when they went outside not a living soul was in sight. Then invisible powers moved pots and pans and turned pictures round on the walls; the door was opened and banged in the middle of the night. According to her there was no other possible explanation but that Grietje was bewitched.

When I asked how and why? I was informed that they had gone to Velddrift to consult the bone-thrower but Grietje had not accompanied them and he had said that she was bewitched. I saw nothing abnormal while there and that evening I told Outa Jantjes about my talk with Grietje's mother.

He was as usual a storehouse of information. According to him the witchcraft and the queer happenings had only started because Grietje's stepfather wanted her to marry one of his crew, and she had set her heart on someone else. It could be that this spirit was protecting Grietje and preventing a marriage to please her father. I could not understand how a spirit could be protecting Grietje by throwing things about.

A few days later however I was fortunate to witness a display of stone throwing. I happened to be fishing off the rocks when I heard people shouting and running. The coloured people were terrified. Stones were raining down from nowhere, mostly pebbles of which there were myriads on the shore near the rocks but this was at least a distance of a hundred yards from the house, whereas the stones appeared to me to have been dropped from the air and not thrown from the ground.

There was not a living soul in the little stone cottage with its one door, kitchen with fireplace and two bedrooms with windows through which one could push a small child with difficulty. Yet from out of this little house pots and pans were being dropped just over the lower closed half of the stable door.

Grietje was there among the crowd very quiet and with a far-away look. Still there was a sort of sly coyness about her when spoken to. Then an Italian fisherman arrived. I knew him well and often sailed with him. He asked me to accompany him into the house which I did. The people outside warned us that "the thing" might attack us. The Italian was a big fellow and I felt quite safe in his strength. Inside the house he made the Sign of the Cross and told me that no evil spirit could venture near when that Sign was made.

There were so many unexplained incomprehensible and mysterious things happening that I was prepared to credit this Sign with the same power. Suddenly all was quiet. No stones fell on the roof, no utensil was moved. We looked everywhere even under the beds. There were five of them. Then as we were standing in the kitchen which also served as a diningroom with its mantel piece covered with paper with frills cut with scissors and decorated with porcelain ornaments and figurines—a little vase lifted itself gently from among all the other ornaments. It floated up to the ceiling, tapped it several times and then suddenly hit the floor at our feet.

My companion leapt over the door and was out. I at least opened the lower door and walked slowly out while my overwhelming impulse was to run away as fast as I could. I was the son of the Seur. Somewhere within me was this command of tradition saying—"Don't be a coward in front of the servants." My mouth was bone-dry and my hair stood on end, but I walked slowly with visibly trembling legs.

I found myself near Grietje and as she raised her eyes to look at me she gave a smile of derision. Now a strange thing happened; my fear gave way to anger and I walked back into the house.

Nothing further happened that day. Some days later there was again some stone throwing and movements of objects and all took place when no physical being could be held responsible. I felt that Grietje knew or was responsible. Perhaps she encouraged this power in order to get her own way.

Then the bone-thrower came while I was not at home or in that area and he burnt powders and drew a circle round the house; drove pegs into the ground and sprinkled some powdery stuff along the circle. He told them to send Grietje away to an aunt in Saldanha Bay so that he could hold the spirit in the circle until Grietje was gone. She left and all the stone throwing stopped. I learned later that the bone-thrower had said that it was not a bad spirit but one who came to help Grietje and that was why he had sent her away. According to her mother the Bushman bone-thrower had said that Grietje had magic power which drew this spirit to her and held him close to her.

Outa Jantjes did not understand this magic power which could draw a spirit to one and hold it close to one to do such things as stone throwing. Years later I saw these manifestations which occurred around Grietje in another light as a mediumistic or psychic phenomena. On reflection it seemed that she somehow enjoyed these manifestations because they could bring her freedom from a stepfather who certainly made life unpleasant for her.

I went to school and seldom saw Outa Jantjes thereafter. His world grew dimmer and dimmer in my mind. New ideas, companions and studies pushed these incomprehensible things of those magical days out of my mind and left them in a slumbering subconscious, only to be awakened by other circumstances of life.

Often in the years that followed I wondered at Outa Jantjes' genius for inventing stories. There was a subtle poetic sense in some of them. One day, while speaking of the silence of the deeply wooded kloofs he told me that this silence was actually made by the spirits who lived there. They sang with the humming insects and the birds but one had to train one's hearing to discern their notes and voices from those of the bees, crickets and birds. Should one walk very silently and not even break a twig and then lie down on your stomach near a little stream or preferably a tiny waterfall under the dense undergrowth, and then listen and listen, one could hear them making tinkling noises like little bits of glass to the accompaniment of the bird songs.

Needless to say I spent several periods lying under the dense bushes trying to hear the song of the spirits of the kloof. And somehow I heard what I sought for the tiny streams made tinkling noises which seemed to harmonise with those emitted by the chorus of insects. No doubt these stories were for my benefit but I also noticed that they formed the topics of their conversation—they could so easily slip over the thresholds of different worlds of images and thoughts.

But the world of the dead played the most prominent part in the minds of old Cape coloured folk of those farm days. To them the next world was populated as this one by a variety of different personalities with different tastes, propensities and temperaments. There were the criminal, the mischievous, the pious and the simple kindly natural spirits.

When I said that we all go to heaven and become angels Outa Jantjes replied that he could not see Outa Willem our shepherd as an angel. Besides if we all became angels why were some of the dead folk whom he knew still roaming around their familiar places trying to do their old jobs not knowing that they have arms of wind. Yet these coloured people formed a sentimental background to our lives. I have seen my father sit up the whole night while an old servant was dying with his head on his lap. There was a strange bond between the master and servant of those semi-feudal days. The Aias carried us on their backs and sang us lullabies at bedtime while the Outas told us stories, mostly of talking animals and I for one enjoyed these thrills of their phantasy world, created with such abundance of vitality and supernormal creatures.

I must mention that during all my childhood years and even to this day I often have dreams of flying. The dream experience was always most pleasant; the feeling of buoyancy; the almost blissful feeling of gliding on and on but making flying movements with my arms. In the dream I made an effort as if swimming in the air. These were propelling movements of the arms and legs, very much the way a frog swims. They have never changed.

Now when I learned of the Bushman's experience—that he visited places in his dreams I also desired to do this but somehow these were always dream places and seldom significant except that the people were people whom I knew on earth. The experience however was so rapturous that I often requested a flying dream in my bedtime prayer. Outa Jantjes said that the Bushman because of his knowledge of magic could travel by means of his spirit which is remembered as a dream which is not full of nonsense.

During 1918 I was a student in Cape Town while the "flu" epidemic was ravaging the country. I contracted it and went through a period when I felt too weak to speak or even swallow. I was told that I had pneumonia but was not delirious. Anyway during this period I had several amazing flying dreams.

On two occasions I found that my companion was a friend who had died when we were round about thirteen or fourteen years of age. I recognized him at once in my dream just as friendly as we had been years before. We flew over mountains and broad valleys but the valleys were unlike those of the Cape—they appeared more like pictures. They were so soft and green—as if they had been laid out by hand. I remembered thinking that I was dead but he assured me that I was not; I was merely on holiday from my sick body and he was showing me the sights of another world where he was learning to make pictures with his mind—even landscapes bigger than any canvas on earth.

When I awoke after this strange dream experience I felt better but inwardly disturbed—life was presenting me with puzzles which I simply could not understand. Was it a mere dream picture of Henry or was it a question of visiting each other in spirit form, as the bone-thrower had said that he could do? All new experiences of a supernormal nature always somehow had a memory link—a mysterious association with the stories which I had heard from Outa Jantjes.

After my recovery I met a lovely Afrikaans girl whose name was Anna. She had such an amazing kindliness about her and such a tremendous affection for animals that it was quite a pleasure to sit in the Botanical Gardens with her and listen to her delightful interpretations of squirrel conversation, and their remarks about humans; and then she told me that she had learned this art from an Outa on their farm who used to regale her as a little girl with stories of animal conversations.

This identification with nature appeared so natural that our metaphors frequently included descriptions of people with animal qualities and peculiarities. But this is not the reason for mentioning my meeting with Anna. She could tell the time correctly when asked at any odd time and during unexpected moments. She just knew.

She could make tables rap and glasses glided from letter to letter spelling out messages. Thereafter we had great fun; a group of boys and girls of from seventeen to nineteen years of age, sitting with our fingers lightly touching the surface of the table while it would rise and tilt in response and tap out the code for yes or no.

Whenever Anna was present the table behaved most animatedly. It would at times tilt so much that it stood on one leg.

Undoubtedly Anna had the power but these qualities and potencies of her person were a secret from her family. "Mammy is sure to think I am possessed by the devil." Then we selected a really heavy table and five of us sat round with the tips of our fingers touching its surface and we obtained faint tappings but when we were joined by Anna this heavy kitchen table rose several inches right off the floor hanging, as it were, from our fingers touching its surface only. We had no physical lifting power that way and yet the table hung for a few moments like a pin from a magnet.

This peculiar power now began to make sense and Anna agreed with me that it was the same power she thought, as that which I had observed in the case of Grietje. But where did this power come from? Apparently it came from our bodies and in particular from Anna's body. She was however a religious girl who always prayed that this power should never be abused.

At times she would sense the illnesses of people and she often described people with a colour emanation. One day while sitting in a tearoom a farmer and his family entered and as the buxom mother and several small children passed our table Anna said : "Oh what a lovely pink colour is oozing from her. That woman has a beautiful mind." And a few moments later there was Anna talking in the most friendly terms to the lady as if they had known each other all their lives.

When I spoke to her about this later she replied that she could never resist the temptation to talk to people whose colours appealed to her and thus flattered me by saying "I like you because of your colours." Her description at the time was a "sort of colour haze" which surrounded each personality. In many cases this was extremely beautiful. Some however were unpleasant and corresponded to their moods and temperaments. She had seen people in their "dorp" going to church in the morning clutching a Bible and hymn books under their arms with colours which showed intense envy, jealousy and hatred.

I learned a great deal from Anna and when I left for Scotland to study medicine she told me never to forget these invisible manifestations because she felt that the day would come when man would understand himself by means of these unknown forces of his being.

During my second year of medicine at Glasgow University I made a friend who had been wounded in the battle of the Somme in September 1918 during the last tremendous onslaught by the British troops. His brother two years older who had been in the same Scottish regiment had been killed. My friend was back at the University to resume his medical studies.

He was interested in psychiatry and took me to Professor Henderson's famous psychiatric clinic where we learned to deal with the remnants of war neuroses and a host of other psychological conditions. In the course of time I expected that somewhere in psychiatry or medicine as a whole I would learn about the powers which I had seen in Grietje and Anna but Freud and Jung could not help, and those with whom I discussed these matters made me feel that they were not respectable subjects from a scientific point of view.

To my surprise my friend Allan shared my views. We were both trying to find the mystery behind physiology and the peculiar physical forces which he had seen operating in a seance given by his Highland landlady. He invited me to his digs to meet this lady. She was a pleasant kindly personality, somewhat plump, round-faced with ruddy cheeks. She had what was colloquially known as "high" colour.

After supper we talked about these matters and she told us how when she first went into service and came to the big city from the north, she discovered her strange powers by knowing what was going to happen beforehand. After a time her mistress consulted her even about racing and she was able to name several winners, but somehow she knew that this was not right as she had been brought up to consider gambling a real sin. Then one day a spirit spoke to her and said his name was Duguid and that he was her guardian.

The lady gave the two of us a trance sitting—the first I had ever attended. It was short but Duguid told me such a great deal about myself and my family that I was most impressed. When I left I wondered : had he read my mind or not? How could a lady with a fairly high-pitched voice imitate a broad Scots voice distinctly masculine?

We discussed this experience with some of our associates and decided to arrange a special seance during which we would investigate this transformation of a female voice into that of a male. My friend Allan made the arrangements and mentioned that the luminous trumpet would be used. He had seen this in one of the private circles for which his landlady was a medium.

On the chosen evening four of us presented ourselves at the lady's apartment which was in a working-class tenement house. One of our party was a complete sceptic and would not accept even an hypothesis that man could possess invisible powers not known to science. Being somewhat under the idealistic influence of the belief that a healthy scepticism was good for science we allowed him to accompany us although Allan said that he believed that antagonistic disbelievers were detrimental to good phenomena.

We arrived to find the lady just finishing washing up the supper dishes so while she was tidying up and preparing herself we had the opportunity to examine the little sittingroom. In one corner was a piano—in another a small table with several photographs of men in uniform. Otherwise the room was cluttered up with enlargements and other family photographs. There was a light in the centre of the room with three electrical bulbs giving a fairly bright light. There was a gramophone with records of sacred music which was played at the beginning of a seance.

There was an eight-inch high trumpet made of cardboard and painted with luminous paint which was plainly visible when the lights were extinguished. We found no hidden wires nor any suspicious device for that matter. The light from the street lamps penetrated the window curtains to some extent and therefore the room although dark allowed a fair amount of dim vision to distinguish the nearby outline of persons and objects.

As our eyes became accustomed to the dark room we could discern objects and movements fairly accurately. The medium was seated about three feet from me. The sceptic sat at the light switch at the door. Allan played the gramophone, a task which he evidently performed on other occasions as the medium insisted that she required the harmony to enter a trance state. She impressed upon us that she felt uneasy as one of us was definitely antagonistic and considered the whole thing absurd. We looked towards the associate at the door but he gave no sign or indication that he felt in any way implicated.

The lights were then extinguished while the gramophone played a hymn sung by some choir. The cardboard trumpet painted with luminous paint stood on a little stool somewhat to the right of the medium. It was plainly visible and although I observed the medium and took careful notice of all her movements and utterances I kept the trumpet in sight all the time.

I could hear the lady trying to make herself comfortable and it appeared as if she were wriggling about in the chair; stretching out her legs and bending her knees; crossing and uncrossing her legs; sighing deeply and yawning repeatedly. Then after a while it was quiet but I felt an icy-cold current of air coming towards me. It seemed to occupy a sort of oblong area around the medium because my friend at the gramophone at the other end of the room and I felt it, while the student on her left and the one at the door did not until much later when it seemed to fill the room, especially when the trumpet was in motion.

It was only a few moments after I made mention of the cold

current of air and my friend affirmed it in his part of the room that a masculine voice spoke in a fairly broad Scottish accent. He said that we could call him Duguid. He was the medium's controlling spirit and guide and mentioned that he had studied medicine in Edinburgh and had passed over in his fifth year in 1900.

He informed us that he knew all about students having been one himself and asked whether we had heard of the Edinburgh landlady who wondered where all the wild students went on graduation day and where the nice young doctors came from. This raised a laugh and we felt more at ease.

Then the voice took on a serious tone and gave us a homely lecture about this new world of knowledge which we were seeking. He pointed out that it was worthwhile to acquaint ourselves with the research that had already been done since all this was part of an unfoldment in the evolution of man to find the interassociation between material and so-called spiritual science. He however preferred to call this aspect of natural knowledge. It was for the science of the future to find the missing links and the gradations.

These words made a profound impression on my mind quite apart from the question as to whether the voice was really what it professed to be or an imitation by the medium. Immediately afterwards as he continued his talk I had reason to doubt the possibility of a conscious impersonation of someone by the medium. He returned to the work on psychic research, and the courage of such men as the late Sir William Crooks, F. W. Meyers, William James and Baron Von Schrenck-Notzing as some of the pioneers in a new field of science.

He also mentioned the name Zoellner and said that we should read his work with the American medium Slade. He impressed on us that the subject of man was indeed a worthy study and that no student could study any subject, arts or science, without a textbook based on the findings of others—the results of their intellectual labours. The student may advance the knowledge and discoveries of his masters but he cannot start *de novo* without availing himself of the storehouse of knowledge accumulated by those inspired by Divine purpose to do so. He insisted that no one should dare to be sceptical to deny and be prejudiced against knowledge of this nature without having first studied the vast literature available.

He said that he knew that we had not made a serious study of the literary evidence. He would strongly advise us to do so. We should be careful not to allow curiosity to make us rush in where angels fear to tread. He was indeed a masterful personality and spoke as if that was his natural voice in contrast to the medium's voice which was somewhat high-pitched.

He said that he would endeavour to move the trumpet but added with a laugh "do not question Jimmie Grey on this force, it is outside his ken." This amused us all because Jimmie Grey was our pet name for Professor Grey who occupied the chair of physics. Soon after this the trumpet, clearly seen by all of us began a swaying movement and gradually it rose higher and higher swerving from side to side as though blown by a breeze, now from this side and now from the other. And then Duguid requested another record; he wanted what he called harmonious vibrations and the trumpet would conduct the choir.

As the record was played the trumpet swept round the room in a wide circle, rising near the ceiling and touching, or tapping it so that we could hear the sounds distinctly. I for one was completely enthralled by this experience for there before my eyes was an energy system at work similar to what I had seen years before in the case of Grietje. Then the trumpet behaved just like a baton —it was conducting the choir. Two of us expressed our amazement when suddenly the room was brightly lit.

The sceptic student at the door had switched on the light because as he admitted afterwards a powerful urge possessed him to do so for he clearly visualized the medium or my friend manipulating the trumpet with a long stiff piece of wire. My eyes were on the trumpet and as the light flooded the room the trumpet did not drop straight down but slid down an invisible incline—that is it came down at an angle to the floor, and hit the small table with photographs of men in uniform and shell ornaments scattering them clattering to the floor.

The whole happening was so unexpected and so sudden that I only thought of the medium when I heard her moaning doubled up in her chair and deathly pale. The ruddy cheeks were gone. Her face and hands were cold and clammy and her pulse was rapid. We carried her to her bedroom and as she retched we were in time with a slop pail. She brought up undigested food and complained of intense colicky pains over her stomach. We obtained some whisky from her neighbour, borrowed hot-water bottles and stayed with her until she was comfortable and the pain had subsided.

By this time her husband had come home and he had every reason to be angry. It took the two of us all our tact and diplomacy to stop him from assaulting our fellow student who had switched on the lights. He did not want to see us again in his house. My friend continued to lodge there and became a member of a closed circle but I although innocent was debarred with the other two.

The following day Allan told me that the lady from across the landing had called him to have a look at the medium's abdomen and he had found a distinct discoloured bruise all over the stomach area—over the location of the solar plexus. The picture was one of blood which had oozed into the tissues. He assured me that his landlady was a sincere, honest and religious woman and she was quite convinced that she had never read books by William James, F. W. Meyers, Sir William Crooks, Baron Von Schrenck-Notzing and Zoellner. She had never heard of these names.

The truth of the matter was that not one of us had any knowledge of these people named. We knew that James was a psychologist but had no idea that he was interested in psychic research. Therefore all these names must have come from Duguid. We made inquiries and were amazed to learn that Zoellner was an astro-physicist who conducted experiments with an American medium called Slade. We found it difficult to deny on the face of all this evidence of ignorance on our part that Duguid was somehow what he claimed to be : an intelligent voice from the dead.

Allan and I could come to no other conclusion but that during the trance a power was emitted by the personality of the medium and that this form of energy was repelled by the artificial light while it was of such an intensity as to be able to be employed for the purpose of movement and levitating the trumpet. We both saw a flimsy cob-web like sort of strand stretching from the medium to the trumpet the moment the lights were turned on.

The bruised condition of her abdominal tissues, exactly over the area of the solar plexus suggested that this concentrated force was driven back into this most important sympathetic plexus of nerves and ganglia and in the process caused a dilatation of blood vessels in that area, draining blood from the head and extremities leaving them cold and clammy while over-stimulating and unbalancing the autonomic nervous system.

The power emitted by Anna in moving the table made one think that somewhere in the human personality there was a function similar to that of an electric conductor. This experience with the Scottish medium therefore had features which were familiar to me and although I was most disappointed that I could not study this lady's powers further I felt sure that we had come across a deeper stratum of human energy and that science had no knowledge of the laws operating in this sphere. In fact it represented a world of energy of a higher order to the grossly physical.

At that time I knew nothing about the mysterious physical phenomena of materialization which occurred during seances given by certain mediums. Ectoplasm was unknown to me and the movements of objects by means of powers known as telekinesis or psychokinesis was not known to me nor did I connect it with the strange behaviour of objects in Grietje's proximity or the power of Anna at table rapping. It was years later when with the immediate pressure of learning medicine having transferred itself to learning from practical experience, with objective and intuitive interpretations, that circumstances directed me to read the work of the men mentioned by Duguid. It was then that I realized that no one could possibly form any idea of psychic phenomena until the works of the pioneers had been studied.

I discovered a monograph by Professor Winther of Copenhagen. He studied a medium, Anna Rasmussen for a number of years. He erected in his laboratory a concrete pillar, I do not know of what size but believe it was quite massive and it stood on a concrete floor. On top of this concrete pillar he fixed a glass chamber of thick glass and in it was suspended a number of pendulums of different lengths and the bobs of which were actually made of different materials. Now comes the amazing part—something proved under the most rigid scientific controls and yet inexplicable by modern science.

Anna Rasmussen would sit not more than three feet away from this contraption and then simply will or wish these pendulums to swing to and fro, change their courses and make them stop to order. She even would will them to knock out the time of day. It was accepted that there was no physical contact between her and the pendulums. Fraud was entirely out of the question and yet the world of science ignored this phenomenon. Was it prejudice or fear because it did not know how to accommodate these supernormal manifestations?

The house of science would have lost its stable foundations if these happenings had to be interpreted by means of the concepts at its disposal. So it was best to ignore it—to deny its presence in the same manner that I found my mind reacted when I could not rationally explain Grietje's ghost. I had formed the theory by that time that the human personality was capable of emitting or radiating a power of an unknown nature. I was influenced in this conception by the visions of colour around people which my little friend Anna perceived and also by that time I had learned that colour and frequency rate of vibration of energy were synonymous.

This conception made me think of the human personality not only in psychological terms but in terms of feelings. At the back of my mind was the subdued impression of some field of force radiating beyond the person and assuming a definite colour pattern to the sight of the clairvoyant. It was fascinating to imagine since I could not see clairvoyantly what the colour surroundings of the people were who consulted me. It made them so much more interesting, and so much more extensive than their mere physical proportions and limitations.

At that time my ideas received strong support when I read of the experiments carried out by Dr. Osty of Paris with the medium Rudi Schneider. His purpose was to discover Schneider's ability to move objects by invisible means some distance from the body. He arranged his experiment so that the object chosen to be moved was protected by an infra-red beam falling on a photo-electric cell. The infra-red beam was considered not to have a repellent effect on this type of energy.

The medium Rudi Schneider went into a trance state. I may add that the arrangement included a device whereby a bell would ring the moment anything obscured the infra-red beam. The bell rang several times and each time it rang an automatic flashlight photograph was taken while the medium remained in deep trance as revealed by the photographs. But the photographs showed no evidence whatsoever of any visible connection between the medium and the bell or the object which was moved. Yet something obscured the infra-red beam and moved the object. Whatever caused this phenomenon was not solid nor was it visible in a flash photograph. Its nature was undoubtedly sensitive to ordinary light and it must have faded away instantaneously the moment the flashlight came on because it did the same while the bell was ringing and ordinary light was shone on the beam.

Dr. Osty then directed his experiment towards the discovery of what the nature of the force was which obscured the infra-red beam and rang the bell, so instead of the bell he employed a quiet period galvanometer and a photographic recording drum. This apparatus would enable the experimenters to observe details of the amazing obscuring factor which moved objects and remained invisible.

But now another surprise awaited them for to their astonishment they found that when the infra-red beam was partially obscured the spotlight of the galvanometer moved exactly at the same rate as the breathing of the entranced medium. This extraordinary manifestation naturally evoked a great deal of interest and was in consequence checked again and again but there it was: the galvanometer recorded the breathing rate of the medium.

The most rational conclusion was that an invisible substance capable of absorbing infra-red light was produced by the medium's body while he was in a deep trance state. This careful scientific experiment revealed that man possessed living forces or systems of energy which as natural components of personality were yet quite unknown to the world of energies which could be radiated from a person under certain conditions.

What role did this energy play between one's will to move an object and the physical movement of one's muscles in the performance of the deed? Any way to my mind it was the same energy as that which produced Grietje's phenomena and moved the table at Anna's touch as well as the trumpet of the Scottish medium. Perhaps the fact that certain people manifested this energy could only mean that it was more loosely integrated with other energy systems in their personalities whereas in most of us this energy is more locked up or more bound in the organism.

The evidence is there that it is not a product of imagination but a fact revealed by psychic phenomena and hence telling a story of our mysterious nature hidden deep beyond the everyday employment of physical energy. Its power to move objects some distance from the body gives one the impression of a radiation of a field of force which even transmitted the vital rhythm of the medium's breathing.

These carefully controlled experiments with Anna Rasmussen and Rudi Schneider not to mention those of the pioneers should leave no doubt in any intelligent and unprejudiced man that we have an unknown mind which reaches deep into all the roots of religion and mysticism. It is almost as if man is invisibly enveloped in power and perceptive faculties which transcend his mundane person. But since by and large most people are uninformed on these matters or have found a certain compensation in aggressive denial that nothing is real or worthwhile outside one's sense world therefore psychic phenomena and the mysterious powers of man are readily rejected.

This I discovered to my dismay and soon learned not to discuss these matters even with people of high intelligence who unconsciously revealed their fascination with the mystic side of life. Even they would want to label me with derogatory terms such as "believing in spooks". Nevertheless looking back over the years it does seem extraordinary how these bits and pieces of supernormal revelations of human power add up to assist the understanding of this puzzle of life.

Starting with the naive conceptions of Outa Jantjes which primarily sensitised my mind for deeper understanding in the years that followed I never really forgot that in this new perspective of man's being my original mentor was Outa Jantjes. Strange people came and told me about mediums and psychic phenomena. I was amazed how with people whom I hardly knew the conversation would enter channels of death and survival or telepathy. I was on most occasions quite sure that I had not initiated this trend of thought. Was there something in my subconscious, some telepathic communication between our beings over and above our commonsense minds? At times I thought so. But Anna had given me the impression that people are drawn together and find their harmonious topics of conversation because of the blending of their colour emanations.

While in my third year of medicine I was doing surgical dressings and writing up case sheets and histories of surgical cases. In the course of my ward visits to patients I met a most cheery young Scots coal miner. The infection of his leg was such that the surgeon had decided to amputate above the knee. Everyone had a greeting for Jamie and his wit and quaint Doric expressions caused roars of laughter. I was drawn to him and would take him cigarettes and other gifts. Furthermore I was learning to speak the dialect and was doing all my history taking where possible in the broad Scots English language. Jamie was very proud of me because of my enjoyment and frequent usage of his native tongue.

Then came the morning of the operation. I was present in the theatre and assisted the anaesthetist beforehand. In those days they employed chloroform and ether and the operating theatres were hot and stifling places with the permeating smell of chloroform and ether. Now it was the usual practice for students sometimes even during their second year to attend operations and it not infrequently happened that the sight of blood and the warm heavy anaesthetic-laden air induced a faint.

The moment we saw a student turn pale, swallow and begin to sway we usually hurried him out to recover in the fresh air. To their credit I must say that I never witnessed a faint where the student did not return to the theatre the moment he had recovered. The sense of shame that one could not stand it and the superior smiles of the nurses constituted a challenge which no budding doctor would evade.

On this particular morning as the saw went through the bone one of the students next to me turned deathly pale and would have fallen as if struck down if I had not caught him and with assistance carried him out into the corridor. In a short while he came to and after swallowing some salvolatile returned to the theatre and stayed there until the operation was completed.

The next day I was accompanying the surgeon on his rounds when we stopped at Jamie's bed and as we moved away he asked me to come round and bring him a few Woodbines his favourite cigarette; besides he had something astonishing to tell me. I duly obtained the cigarettes and listened to Jamie's most extraordinary experience.

He said that shortly after he started to breathe the anaesthetic he found himself somewhere near the ceiling of the room looking down at us giving him chloroform and ether. He then followed the body into the theatre and saw the operation. He thought that he was dead and said to himself: "Michty me there is nae punishment for ma sins." But while he was up there above our heads he saw a student faint and as we carried him out of the theatre he also saw a gossamer-like translucent form of the student walking out with us; in fact accompanying his physical body. Thereafter everything went black and he remembered no more until he regained consciousness from the anaesthetic.

This amazing story was extremely convincing because I could not find anyone who had talked to Jamie about the student who had fainted; besides Jamie had a fair amount of pain and was hence given sedatives and so slept most of the time. I had at that stage of my experience no knowledge of the existence of what is known as an astral body. This incident occurred some years before Sylvan Muldoon and Hereward Carrington published *The Projection of the Astral Body*.

Outa Jantjes had of course told me of a spirit body but although I associated this possibility with religious beliefs it somehow was not sufficiently substantial and tangible for my intellect to view it as a practical factor—an actual inner component that could perceive and remember events when the brain was unconscious and even narcotised.

Jamie however insisted that he was wide awake in his astral body and after his first realization that he could see his own body with the surgeon at work he felt delightfully free and contented; in fact he was quite indifferent to his body. He thought that he had died under the anaesthetic. He then confessed to me that it was not the operation which he had dreaded for he knew Mr. McEwan was a brilliant surgeon, but the anaesthetic. He had always had a terrible fear of an anaesthetic and suffocation since he had had his tonsils removed as a small boy. He told me almost in a whisper that he made jokes and laughed to keep this fear from overwhelming him. Therefore whenever he closed his eyes he just kept on praying that God should prevent him from making a fool of himself by starting to scream and struggle the moment the mask was put on his face. It would have been too awful to live down such a shameful exhibition when everyone was so kind to him, especially the nurses.

But as I was present at the induction of the narcosis I remembered him as smiling and being quietly co-operative. He admitted that a calm resignation had come over him and he had felt that this life was not the be-all and end-all of existence.

A few months after his discharge Jamie came back for an artificial limb but he complained of a phantom leg and foot. He could feel pain in this non-existent leg and the pressure of the bed clothes on the invisible toes. He said that the phantom leg was a nuisance for sometimes he would forget his crutch and step off the chair on the phantom leg and land on the floor. The surgeons considered operating on the nerve endings in the stump. They thought the phantom was a mental production set up by sensations coming from these nerve endings and ascending to his brain. In the end Jamie refused an operation; he would rather have a phantom leg than face another anaesthetic.

It is not appropriate to enter into the many theories about phantom limbs and the idea that they result from a persistence of the body image in the mind of the patient. Many different operations have been performed for this condition on the spinal cord and the brain and often these were not successful whereas in others the phantom disappeared by itself.

Now at that time as I have mentioned I had no knowledge of the astral body nor of the literature on the subject. Jamie however put a suggestion into my mind. He said that he had given this invisible limb a great deal of thought while spending his days at his mother's cottage somewhere in Lanarkshire. He reasoned that when he found himself out of his body in the operating theatre he was sure that he had a body and limbs and when we carried the unconscious student out of the theatre his phantom body was walking alongside and it had limbs although it glided rather than walked. Therefore if there were this phantom body, which no one could persuade him was not so, then this phantom body could quite easily continue to have a limb even after the physical leg had been removed, and he thought that what he felt was the leg of this phantom body.

With the growth of knowledge on astral projections and phantoms produced from thoughtforms I found it very difficult to dismiss as unworthy of consideration Jamie's theory about his phantom leg. Maybe there are astral limbs which continue to influence consciousness because of the relationship of the different dimensionalities of energy which make up the human personality. We have no scientific knowledge of the peculiar constitutions and biochemical integrations which produce trance mediums, telekinesis, ectoplasm and astral projections automatically and at will.

Medical psychology will have to make room for these facts of psychic research and, as I see it, we might have to accept the astral body as a working hypothesis from which we should proceed to understand the different invisible substantialities of man. The exclusion of the findings of psychic research, especially with regard to astral travel and ectoplasmic materializations, from our scientific concepts of man has I think precluded psychiatry and philosophy from presenting us with evidence for an ultimate psychic unity of man.

Under these circumstances we have to ask ourselves from a scientific angle whether we are really capable of valuing man's ideals and aspirations? When the human mind reveals power entirely different from the sense perception with which we have learned to understand our world and our fellowmen then it is necessary for us to reach out for knowledge about these faculties which have in the past been buried deep under layers of superstition, magical ideas and practices of naive primitive mentalities.

Having been labelled with these stigmas of degeneracy, our civilization has as yet not truly valued the faculties of extrasensory perception. The powers of the human mind such as telepathy, clairvoyance and precognition alone are quite different from our usual way of acquiring memories from sense perception. They decidedly tell a story which imply that our ideas of time and causation are relative to the world of our senses. Therefore these ESP faculties have transcendent powers and means of obtaining knowledge. Here there is a challenge to the intellect capable of an unprejudiced rational approach to these mysterious resources associated with the mind of man.

CHAPTER II

UNKNOWN SYSTEMS OF ENERGY

It was the month of February in the Tulbagh valley thirty years ago to be exact. The presentations of that morning were like many other mornings at that time of the year.

Always there were the azure skies with far-distant fleecy clouds, all merging heaven with the blue towering grandeur of the Winterhoek mountains; while down below in the valley the simmering heat of the early day brought out the chorus of humming bees and insects in that arcadian land of fruit and wine. I was in general medical practice at the time.

We had brought out our favourite West Highland terriers from Scotland and I was enjoying myself playing with them on my lawn before going my rounds, when a young coloured man jumped off a foaming horse and implored me to come to his father whom he had left as dead. They lived in a coloured hamlet a few miles from the village.

I learned from him that his father had been sick for a few weeks and had the fever. He was being attended by my colleague who at that moment was away in the district on an urgent call. The patient apparently had collapsed as a result of a haemorrhage from the bowel. I surmised that it was a case of typhoid fever.

On arrival I found an emaciated body—almost skin and bone whose heart sounds fluttered faintly. He was unconscious and did not respond to touch or the spoken word. Even the difficulty of introducing a needle into the almost invisible and collapsed veins caused no physical reaction. Only the fluttering heart sounds told the tale that life was hanging on to a body by a tiny thread.

Saline and glucose were given into the vein and other cardiac stimulants. After some time the pulse became fuller, the beats slowed down a bit and the pulse felt more powerful. The breathing became less shallow and moved the chest wall which it had only done faintly before the saline and glucose flowed into the vein.

Then his eyelids fluttered and feebly opened as little slits through which he peeped at me. He sighed once or twice and the lids closed again. His pulse was now steadier and there were signs that no more blood was being passed.

I decided to return again that evening and left. I was busy as typhoid was quite prevalent at that time of the year. Late that afternoon I visited him again. He had taken nourishment and there was no further haemorrhage. The patient was eager to talk to me but I persuaded him to wait a day or two.

He continued to improve according to the messages which they sent me but he wanted to tell me something very important, though as I had handed the case over to my colleague I had to make arrangements to visit him again to hear what he so eagerly wanted to tell me. As I stopped my car in the shade of a tree his wife came hurriedly to meet me and somewhat excitedly told me that her husband wanted to send for the minister so that he could be present when he told me what had happened to him during the time that his body had been unconscious.

This story immediately aroused my interest and after several years the experience of Jamie came vividly back to me because she told me that her husband had known of everything that had taken place during the time when I was finding it so very difficult to introduce a needle into his vein.

When I entered his room he was so excited that he wanted to sit up. He felt that his experience was absolute proof of his religion and that as an elder in the Mission Church he wanted to tell his minister and the whole congregation that there was no death of the spirit. I had some difficulty in restraining him, and feared a delirious excitement as a result of his toxic condition but he had to tell me in his expressive Afrikaans with the appropriate gestures. He said that when I found his body unconscious, near dead or dying, he was wide awake and was never more alive in all his life.

It had all started by him beginning to feel light-headed and dizzy. He tried to look at his wife and children but they were blurred and then it felt as if he were floating or drifting; anyway the sensation was very pleasant. He felt as light as a feather and then he looked down and saw his miserable physical body lying on the bed. He said that he felt disgusted when he thought of the man he was in the days when he had handled a brown mule team, the pride of the Swartland.

He decided that he must have died and found himself floating on air out of the house. His motion was very much like what he had experienced in a fast train when it had seemed as if the train stood still and the telegraph poles were going past. He saw his son on horseback but he went ahead of him and he knew that his son was going to call Dr. Ritter but he gained the impression that the doctor was not at home.

How he knew these things he did not say. He then found himself at my house and saw me rolling a ball along the lawn which was chased by little white dogs. He had never seen dogs like those before but immediately recognized them as being of the same species as the white doggie on a whisky bottle.

Then he went back to look for his son Hendrik and saw how he was treating the poor horse in order to make it gallop faster. He shouted to Hendrik not to ride the horse in that manner but somehow he was not heard and made no impression on Hendrik. He was sure that he was dead and wondered what would happen next.

He decided to visit his friends at Wolseley and straight away he went there. He tried to talk to them but they did not hear him. In fact they seemed to walk right through him. He then decided to go to Ceres to visit people there but a strange power pulled him back to his home. There he saw me arriving.

He watched how I examined his heart and then hang a glass jar on a nail above his bed. He saw me tie a band round his arm and how I rubbed and rubbed the arm looking for a vein before putting a needle into his arm. He also noticed the perspiration on my forehead and face; I took my jacket off and hung it over a chair. Then I connected a rubber-tube to the needle.

His wife came in with cloths soaked in brandy to place over his heart. He noticed my expression as I waved her away. He also knew that those brandy cloths would not bring him back. Why should he come back when he felt so well, so free and so exhilarated? He was sure that he had left his body for good but somehow he had a feeling that he was still attached to his body.

He was quite sure that he felt a queer throbbing as if a pulse were beating all through his new and invisible body and then his mind went blank. But before this happened he knew that I was trying to bring him back to his earth life and he did not want to return. When asked whether he did not think of his wife's grief and sorrow if he had left this world he answered that in reality he felt so fine that he did not give their earthly cares a thought. He however felt a sense of annoyance at my persistence to get the fluid into his body.

After his mind went blank he came to in his body and it felt as heavy as lead. All the power of buoyancy and freedom was gone. He was conscious of extreme exhaustion with hardly the power to breathe.

He tried to look at me to make sure that he was in his body but the memory of his experience of having been outside his body was something so real, so vivid and in such detail that he had no doubt that during that time he had been in a spiritual body.

When asked why as a religious man he had not immediately thought of heaven seeing that he thought he was dead he answered that such a thought never entered his mind. He was more interested in what other people were doing and especially in the amazing power of travelling wherever he wanted to be until some mysterious force pulled him back to his home and his old body.

Since this time Muldoon's book on the astral self has appeared in many editions and there have been many others who have had similar experiences. To my mind this patient's story was not an invention, neither a dream nor an hallucination. He was not the class of person who would have invented such a story; besides the clarity of detail and the descriptions of his feelings and sensations away from his body had a unique element of freedom about them which people in astral projections usually claim.

The one factor of importance which I was assured he was never told of by his son was my playing with my West Highland terriers. He described my rolling the tennis ball for them to chase; now by the time his son came to call me I had stopped throwing the ball and was in fact merely fondling my doggies. The rolling of the ball was therefore an incident which he had seen while in his astral state.

Since that time I have come across other experiences which could only be explained by accepting the hypothesis of travelling in the astral form. The important factor in these experiences is the existence of an inner body—evidently quite substantial but of a much finer and tenuous substance. Jamie said it was translucent and gossamer-like.

The typhoid patient made an interesting observation : that the people whom he saw when out of his body all had a sort of cloudy material around their bodies and these were of different colours. He did not observe these carefully but remembered this haziness of different colours surrounding the people. I attached a great deal of importance to this observation because clairvoyants claim to see these auras of people and I am quite sure that this simple coloured man had never heard of an aura.

He in any case denied ever having had such an idea in his mind. His experience hence fits in with what clairvoyants consider a natural component of the astral body. It rather lends support to the notion that clairvoyance means seeing with the consciousness and visual faculty of the astral body. Hence the world of second sight could be said to belong to this inner personality known as the astral. We shall have more to say about this at a later stage.

In our physical bodies we are children of time, space and matter and our minds have grown up accustomed to this perspective; it is therefore very difficult for us to accept another world not bound by the limitations and frontiers of commonsense.

But we do receive a certain amount of encouragement from the physicists—perhaps not directly and intentionally but by presenting us with thoughts for enlarging our comprehension—especially the world of protons, electrons and neutrons for instance, they do give us a perspective very different from that of our sense experience because we do not directly apprehend these elements as part of our physical world.

Man had existed for untold ages before electrons and protons entered his universe of thought; although therefore the physicists gave us a picture of a world made up of these fundamental constituents they also informed us that these little bricks with which they built our world could change and become waves of energy. Indeed all things in our physical world are built up on positive and negative charges with rapid motion and radiation and absorption of radiation.

It does seem as though the science of physics has been preparing our minds, albeit unwittingly, to become accustomed to new values and to seek beyond the sense world for a deeper reality. Both Jamie and the coloured typhoid patient apparently slipped out of the system of energy of one dimensionality into another and felt quite at home.

Let us assume that those two experiences of the Ego being conscious out of the physical body are essentially the truth then it should be self-evident that our knowledge of human physiology is most rudimentary. It would hence be of extreme importance in our search for knowledge of the personality to ascertain whether such an entity as the astral body is really a vital component of man.

For once its presence is established many other problems belonging to extrasensory perception should fall away. It is of importance therefore to form a clear conception of what is so far known about the astral body and to find a place for it in our understanding of supernormal phenomena. Many have written on the subject of astral projection and the ability to retain an enhanced consciousness when far distant from the physical body. I shall here however draw from Sylvan Muldoon and Hereward Carrington's book on "The Projection of the Astral Body."

I consider that Muldoon's experiences are most enlightening and his deductions and theories constructive and logical, and of a higher order than mere attractive plausability. His knowledge must be accepted as based on fact; when one studies his experiences one can hardly doubt the vital role of an astral body. I would strongly recommend anyone who is desirous of a more profound understanding of man's nature to read this work, characterised by its honesty and sincerity.

The astral is defined as the double of the physical body. It resembles the physical and normally coincides with it cell for cell. It consists of a more tenuous substance which is capable of increasing and lowering its rate of vibration. It can become of such a high frequency rate of vibration that it can pass through physical human beings and find no obstruction anywhere, and it can reach a degree of lowered vibration when it is almost solid and unable to pass through certain forms of matter.

It is also capable of condensing energy in these lower frequency rates to the extent of moving physical objects. Normally it is an inner being of one's outer physical being. Its composition is said to be a semi-fluid or subtle form of matter invisible to the naked eye. The astral can be understood as more truly the real man than the physical, but it in turn is the outer body of a still more inner Ego and being; that inner-self of man which is known as the soul or true psyche.

The Biblical reference to these inner degrees of being and consciousness is clearly presented by Paul in 1 Corinthians 15, verses 44, 46, 50 and 51, as follows : "It is sown a natural body, and it is raised a spiritual body. There is a natural body, and there is a spiritual body." "Howbeit that was not first which is spiritual, but that which is natural, and afterward that which is spiritual."

My interpretation of Paul's exposition signifies that man came into the world with the spiritual as the invisible inner and had to shed the first body, the natural and physical one, to attain the spiritual. By "natural" he no doubt intended to convey the idea of belonging to the physical dimension of existence, namely the earth life.

He went on and said : "Now this I say brethren that flesh and blood cannot inherit the Kingdom of God, neither does corruption inherit incorruption." Again he emphasized that in the next life there cannot be the outer matter of flesh and blood and certain components of man will have to be shed.

Then he came to the part of this transition and the dynamics of a new vehicle of consciousness. He said : "Behold I show you a mystery; we shall not all sleep, but we shall all be changed." This could mean that after death some might sleep or remain unconscious of their new environment for a time but each and everyone shall attain a new body. Paul must have had profound knowledge of psychic matters. He said in I Corinthians 2, verse 10 : "But God hath revealed them unto us by his spirit; for the spirit searcheth all things, yea, the deep things of God."

His reference to different types of matter and his emphasis on physical bodies and ethereal bodies, becomes very significant when we think in terms of vehicles of the Ego with the astral as the inner of the physical. In I Corinthinans 15, verses 39 and 40 he illustrates this point of various forms of substantialities as vehicles of consciousness as follows : "All flesh is not the same flesh : but there is one kind of flesh of men, another flesh of beasts, another of fishes, and another of birds." Hence even in the world of physical material for forming bodies there is a diversity of matter.

"There are celestial bodies, and bodies terrestrial, but the glory of the celestial is one, and the glory of the terrestrial another." I do not think that Paul meant celestial bodies to refer to heavenly bodies such as stars and planets. I think that he elaborated his theme about man possessing bodies other than the physical, and that his reference to celestial bodies could be interpreted as ethereal bodies relative to the forms of physical matter. I think that Paul clearly established the fundamental principle that man has more than one dimensionality of being.

If one reads Muldoon and then Paul one will find that the New Testament teems with psychic experiences and phenomena and that the astral body played a prominent part on some dramatic occasions. It seems quite reasonable to accept that the astral body itself forms the vehicle for a more inner degree of Ego and consciousness, known as the Soul. The bodies hence become more and more celestial to use Paul's term, in comparison with the now terrestrial or earthy.

To return to the astral in its interassociation with the life in physical matter, we are informed that during our full waking activities the astral body is in complete coincidence with the physical body. The one fits into the other, like a hand into a glove in all movements and actions. But when we sleep a change occurs and the astral moves out of coincidence. It might withdraw not more than an inch from its usual anchorage in the physical cells and nerves.

During these periods a good clairvoyant might see it very little out of its usual identical position, or it might be seen as hovering just above the sleeper. If one for instance sleeps on one's stomach the astral would be in a position with its face down and also suspended as if lying on its stomach. The same would happen if the sleeper lies on his back or side. The astral takes up the same position.

Whilst in a faint, or suffering from concussion, in a trance state or under an anaesthetic the astral similarly withdraws from the physical body. I suppose this occurs in all cases of unconsciousness. When the astral withdraws under the above conditions inclusive of sleep then the projection is known by such terms as automatic, spontaneous or involuntary separation of the astral body.

Some people have a peculiar constitutional make-up which facilitates astral projection in a voluntary manner as a result of concentrated self-training, as in the case of Muldoon. On such occasions the astral completely leaves the physical and travels to far distant places with a delightful airborne freedom and with an Ego keenly alert; indeed at a high pitch of clear consciousness.

The person could as a result of an accident, narcosis, sleep or unconsciousness due to illness and exhaustion come to himself in his astral body as Jamie and the coloured typhoid patient experienced. He could, I daresay, travel around at will until the will of self-preservation and the pull of vital forces compel return to the body.

Now the mystery of this process of returning to the body and one's attachment to the body is contained in the astral cable or silver cord of the Bible. We read in Ecclesiastes XII, 6 and 7: "The silver cord be loosened and the golden bowl be broken." This is a description of the process of death for the next verse states: "Then shall the dust return to the earth as it was, and the spirit shall return unto God who gave it."

Muldoon believes that this cord is attached to the back of the head—that portion of the brain known as the medulla oblangata—the house of vital centres. It could leave the body at the front, the side or the back of the head depending on the position of the physical body at the time of the projection. Not only does the cord participate in the projection but it has been described as being composed of the same sort of substance as the astral body.

But no one knows where the cord comes from and where it goes once the bodies are in coincidence again. Muldoon states that its elasticity is far beyond imagination; in fact there is no known material with the stretching qualities of the astral cord. It always stretches from the astral to the physical body as long as there is life in the physical. Only death severs it as mentioned in Ecclesiastes.

The nearer the astral body is to the physical the greater is the thickness of the cord and the greater its magnetic pull. Muldoon states that when the astral body is slightly out of coincidence the cord is as thick as the diameter of an American silver dollar but at this thickness it also has an aura extending about six inches around it.

Therefore the astral or silver cord is highly vitalized for it has an active electro-magnetic radiation which can be seen as a luminosity surrounding it when the cord is at its maximum diameter or when the two bodies, astral and physical, are close together. But as the bodies separate farther and farther apart, the cord decreases in thickness and begins to stretch into infinity. Ultimately it is as thin as a sewing thread and then over very long distances it can only be seen by the astral personality as a single strand of a cobweb.

How apt is the description which our language has evolved

from unconscious knowledge when it says "life hangs on a thread." According to Muldoon health plays an important role because health means that a great deal of energy is stored in the astral body and hence the flow of energy through the cord will be stronger and so the cord's activity could extend over long distances. There is more power at the disposal of the astral body to roam about within other domains, terrestrial or astral. But it is also true that the more energy stored in the astral the greater the health and this implies that the astral body under these conditions is more adherent to the physical and will not move out of coincidence easily.

We can now understand what happened to the typhoid patient and in unconsciousness with shock or narcosis as in the case of Jamie. These patients never mentioned the astral cord; I suppose they were not conscious of it as they had their minds occupied in other directions and since both thought they were dead this might have affected their astral perceptions. Muldoon considers the astral body the condenser of cosmic energy which gives us animation and power.

There is a range or distance known as "cord activity"; this distance corresponds with the health of the individual and in Muldoon's case varied according to his health from eight to fifteen feet. At this distance one could feel a pulsating action with expansion and contraction; the throb of the heart could be felt in the astral body and was expressed through the cord. Each breath taken in the astral could be seen pulsing over the astral cord to cause a similar reaction in the body. Muldoon found that when he breathed deeply in the astral body a short distance from his physical the pull on the cord increased drawing the astral back into the physical body.

Any emotion similarly will increase the pull of the cord and draw one back to the body—fear is especially prone to do this. The emotions increase the heart-beat and this in turn pumps more vital forces into the cord and so it shortens and pulls the astral back into coincidence. Muldoon considers that the force in the cord remains mysterious. At times it projects the astral phantom or body steadily and at other times erratically, throwing it to one side or the other. It is not the phantom which moves itself but this subconscious force in the cord.

Once the astral body is outside the range of cord activity it is free and only acts to its own will but all the time there flows this cosmic energy from the astral body or phantom along this single thread or strand of a cobweb to the physical body. Although at that distance one is selecting and following your own wishes, where you want to go and so on nevertheless there is a subconscious intelligence fully aware of the situation and it brings you back whether you want to or not when it considers that it is time to return and occupy the physical body.

Even from these brief glimpses which I have mentioned one cannot deny that there is a great field for science concerned not only with the astral body itself but with the extraordinary control and energy and its interchange that takes place through the silver cord. These mysterious perspectives loom up whenever we begin to think beyond the limits imposed by our physical bodies. Man is undoubtedly a manifold of energy systems. It seems as though he is a building, consisting of several storeys with a single Ego having a consciousness for each floor and each floor being the substance of the dominant energy system operating there and limiting the vision and perspective of the central Ego.

Always there is some insulation between the floors so that consciousness cannot easily slip over into the one above or below. Even in our physical world there appears to be a spectrum of energy at the disposal of life. We have learned from the physicists that energy moving at different rates of frequency of vibration gives us the difference between one object and another. This is almost stating in scientific terms what Paul said in 1 Corinthians, Chapter 15.

We can then accept on scientific grounds that there is a principle of varying frequency of vibrations from the most solid through water, steam, heat and light to worlds of activity beyond the range of our sense experience or perceptions. For instance our vision stops at violet and ultraviolet is invisible, and so we find a whole series of rates of vibrations or radiations like X-rays, gamma-rays and cosmic-rays which form the shortest waves of our electromagnetic spectrum.

All these invisible vibrations of energy give rise to realities which our ordinary consciousness cannot register. Now we might well ask : is it rational to assume that this spectrum of energy which is a constituent of the cosmos and which gives us a perspective of its various strata of activity, movement and change stops at the cosmic rays? Is it not more probable that we have only discovered some of the lowest steps of the ladder and that the spectrum continues progressively on into eternity?

Perhaps its next phase is the energy system forming the silver cord of the astral body and then the energy system with its scale of vibrations forming the astral body proper, and from there the next system of psyche or soul frequencies on into the dizzy heights of thought.

The knowledge which we have acquired from those who have experienced astral projection or consciousness in the astral body has shown that the cord behaved as an intelligence. It would resist projection according to certain laws and promote it according to others. Conflicting forces could be brought into operation by certain conditions. Even when the astral phantom, with its intellect and consciousness was miles away from the body, exploring some place or other and the cord was a mere thickness of one strand of a cobweb it could pull the astral back and plunge it into the body with a sensation which was said to be unpleasant and repercussive.

It is fascinating to ask : what is the intelligence behind the astral cord? What intelligence will operate and control these movements? Before one ventures an answer to these questions it is necessary to observe that the consciousness which the Ego experiences in the astral body is of a much higher, clearer and alert nature than that known in the brain state. They are said to perceive aesthetic qualities and colours which our sensory intellects cannot apprehend. The astral has therefore a consciousness of a finer quality as if it were a little transcendent to the sensory consciousness of our terrestrial bodies.

But there is evidence that the astral consciousness has an unconscious will which operates according to certain laws and can cut short the will and purpose of the astral conscious mind. Let us assume that this unconscious will of the astral is actually the deeper layer of the Ego for which the astral is a mere vehicle, but a vehicle of a higher order than the physical body. This unconscious will of the astral shows that it has greater command and control of the energy systems making up the spectrum of the being than any other level of consciousness.

It is reasonable to assume that this greater intelligence and power operating the forces of life is the soul of man itself. The silver cord is to my mind an intermediate energy substance between the astral system and the electronic nature of the cells of the physical body. The silver cord could be a condensed or concentrated energy force being primarily the radiations of nerve fibres, nerve sheaths, nerve plexuses and ganglia of the central nervous system. It could be drawn from all over the body to the main nuclei and vital centres of the midbrain and medulla oblongata and from here assume a cord-like appearance to the astral sight but remain magnetically in association with the bioelectric system of the physical body. In other words, it still has its electromagnetic roots in the molecules and atoms of the body.

The break has to take place here within the cells of the physical body because apparently the moment these cells cannot generate sufficient energy to hold this magnetic nerve current then death occurs and the astral floats away. Perhaps this neuric or nerve cell radiation is the true source of ectoplasm which trance mediums produce for materializations. Maybe it is the system of energy which heals wounds and brings about healing in general. So one can imagine different frequencies of rates of vibration forming different systems of energy with thought as the highest or the supreme power of the human psyche.

But thought itself will only be able to control and direct these systems of energy if it operates under conditions where this energy is in abundance and free from the restrictions or resistances of the magnetic pull of lower rates of vibration. Hence there have to be people in whom these interassociations of energy systems are loose and in whom disintegration of a partial nature is possible to produce the vast range of physical phenomena credited to mediums of the past such as those employed by Dr. Glen Hamilton and before that time Eusapia Palladino, the famous Eva C., Rudi Schneider and many others.

Did the Scottish landlady control the energy system which moved the trumpet with her own astral mind or perhaps her soul consciousness? or was it the will and consciousness of Duguid in his astral personality? Was it the medium's mind or Duguid who manipulated this energy system radiated by her and forming the strands which moved the trumpet?

It is necessary to elaborate on the preceding factors to show that the consciousness after death can retain intentions formed during life and seriously make an attempt to execute these as physical acts. During my student years in Scotland there occurred the great railway strike. A period almost of a national crisis coupled with large-scale unemployment and disgruntled men on the dole. It so happened that hooligan elements and professional beggars on several occasions rang doorbells and then forced their way into homes resulting in robberies by force. The Police Chief issued a press warning to citizens not to open their doors in response to the bell until they had first ascertained who the caller was.

I was then engaged to my wife and frequently called at their home on my way from hospital in the evenings. I therefore arranged not to ring the bell but to give three characteristic knocks; two firm and loud knocks followed by a pause and then the third knock. This method of announcing myself was soon adopted by my wife's mother and thereafter even long after the crisis we continued to announce ourselves, even to our friends by means of our knocks.

Then a few years later when my wife and I were leaving Scotland for South Africa my wife's mother and I were alone one evening while she played my favourite pieces on the piano. After a while we talked about our departure and how much she was going to miss my wife. At that moment the idea came into my mind to ask her to enter into a promise that should she die before me she would attempt at all costs to give the three knocks in my presence. After some days I plucked up courage to speak to her about this idea of knocking after death. At first she did not like the idea at all and felt that it would make her conscious of something morbid.

But a few days before we sailed I again broached the subject but this time I emphasized that such an experience from either of us would, at least to the one physically alive leave no doubt about the possibility of surviving death with intentions formed during earth life. She agreed very solemnly to remember this as a promise and to give these knocks as clearly as possible should she pass over before me and I was to do the same should I leave this world before her.

Six years later I was working in the Union Mental Service at a hospital in Cape Town. My wife's mother was well and we received weekly letters from her in Glasgow. At that time mail took about twenty-one days between the Cape and Scotland. On the evening of the 14th February 1931 I came home from the Psychiatric Juvenile Court Clinic feeling indisposed with a mild attack of influenza. I went to bed without dinner and dosed myself so as to be able to do at least twenty lumbar punctures the next morning as part of a research project. There was no one who could do the work for me at that time.

I awoke about five o'clock on the morning of February 15th. I found my temperature normal and I had a healthy hunger. I therefore went to the pantry and made myself a light breakfast. Thereafter I went to lie on my bed in my dressing gown to read the *Cape Argus* which I had not read the previous evening. I looked through the window and outside the long beams of the summer sun were sweeping across the Cape Peninsula. Now I must mention that my bedroom door opened on to a passage which ran the length of the house next to its front wall. My wife had her own room next to mine and our sons were sleeping in the room next to hers.

I was lying on the bed smoking a cigarette and engrossed in the paper when I was startled by two loud knocks inside my bedroom door which was shut, there was a distinct pause and then came the third loud knock. By this time I was off my bed and had jerked open the door. But there was no one in the passage. All the outside doors were locked and the gauze frames over the open windows were firmly secured as protection against mosquitoes from the Liesbeek river.

As I opened my bedroom door my wife who was awake called out to ask what the knocks were. Now let me describe my feelings on that occasion just as I wrote them down after returning to my room to reflect on the event. The moment the knocks were given I was instantly conscious of the presence of my wife's mother. I knew that she had died and I knew that she was in my room. Although I rushed to examine the doors and windows and even went into the garden I did all that to exclude any argument that someone could have given the knocks and escaped.

As I heard the knocks I felt a wave of gladness. There was animation and joyousness in the immediate atmosphere. I was keenly aware of her presence; indeed it was physically palpable. Hers was a jubilant presence as though our very souls were embracing each other with delight. Our experiment or test had proved a success. She had produced evidence that a promise made during life if intently and sincerely desired could be carried into effect after death. The will and the intention went over in the same psyche. Indeed the psyche had a consciousness which could carry intention, memory and desire over from one life into another.

The idea that she had died and that grief and sorrow should be the natural reactions did not seem to have any significance for me during those moments. Actually I gained the impression that inwardly the two of us were on an island in a sea of humanity and around us were the barriers of man's psychic limitations. I tried to reach her being telepathically. There was so much that I wanted to know but all that registered in my mind were impressions which I could be said to have imagined. I gained these thought impressions as decided and positive. I felt that she had passed over only a few moments before giving the knocks and that her power for staying in this sphere was fading because there was a gravitational pull of the other sphere of existence.

The knocks were only possible because of her intense desire to inform us of her death and because she could draw on a power emitted from my body and in conjunction with which she could manage to make the knocks as loud as possible. The fact that my wife heard them eliminated the possibility of my being accused of having had an hallucination.

I was sitting on my bed when these impressions transpired and felt actually elated as if some wonderful experiment had been a success. I was oblivious to the fact that somehow I had to break the news to my wife and that her grief would be great. The departure of her mother's presence was perceived by my feelings. I did not think but could almost feel her being receding away from me as if drawn away into eternal disappearance. I was standing on the quayside of life watching a departure by means of feelings.

Now it was about five-thirty on the morning of Tuesday the 15th of February 1931 that my wife and I distinctly heard the three knocks just as her mother used to give them in Glasgow. That day passed and although I made several inquiries no cablegram had arrived. Neither on the Wednesday, Thursday or Friday did we hear anything but I never doubted the experience and felt convinced that my wife's mother had died and had given the knocks as proof of her life after death.

Then came Saturday morning. I was in the wards when I received a telephone call to the effect that a cablegram from overseas was awaiting me at the office. The cablegram was from my wife's sister and it read—"Mother passed away this morning, pneumonia," and the date was the 15th February. It was a deferred cablegram and had been held up along the line. This simple experience carried such conviction for me that I could not think of any argument which could demolish this subjective and objective confirmation of life's continuation.

During 1941 I met Mrs. Shearer in whose presence strange phenomena had taken place during trance states and also on other occasions when she was not in a trance. I studied her mediumship for over fourteen years and found that she displayed a variety of psychic manifestations, except materializations. I was particularly interested in the physical effects which were of the poltergeist type of phenomena as well as the exalted ethical dissertations in Elizabethan English during her trance states. But more of this later.

Mrs. Shearer is Jewish and belongs to the Hebrew religion. The testimonies of the most reliable witnesses conveyed the impression that she was noted for her charm, warm-heartedness and generosity. She loved acting and her great ambition was the stage. She excelled in elocution and dramatic performances and was especially outstanding in reciting Shakesperian works. Her father had the same psychic abilities and was fairly good at obtaining telepathic impressions. He was also a great practical joker. Fun and amusement were some of his chief preferences. In fact most members of this family have this ability to clown and play the fool.

Mrs. Shearer showed a complex personality : fun, practical jokes, hoaxes, mimicry, mime and impersonations were the order of the day even during business hours. As a girl she displayed a peculiar fondness for the scholarly company of senior men. She married early and her stage ambitions could not be fulfilled. At the age of twenty-one she had a baby eighteen-months old and with her baby was staying at her mother's home while her husband was away on business. She and her baby shared a large room with her sister and a cousin. Being in the mood for playing pranks and jokes with the intention of frightening the others she professed to see a ghost standing near the door.

The other two became frightened and huddled together. To increase their fear Mrs. Shearer pulled their blankets at which they screamed believing that some supernatural force was at work. But while Mrs. Shearer was busy making suggestions to increase their discomfort things suddenly began to happen. Electric light bulbs left their sockets and crashed with loud reports on the floor. Picture frames moved and turned over on the walls. Combs, brushes, under-clothes and odds and ends went flying all over the room. Her mother heard the commotion and came upon a scene of disorder.

Mrs. Shearer had no power to stop the invisible movement of objects and her mother being by this time also upset at the mysterious activities of objects stayed the night with them. But the baby slept peacefully through all the commotion and noise. Mrs. Shearer's late mother was one of the most sincere, honest, kind, truthful and noble persons I have ever known. There were no embellishments of her thoughts. She was always the audience before whom some of her children acted out their fanciful pranks and mimicry.

The day after the nocturnal disturbance, objects were occasionally seen to fall down from their places or move when Mrs. Shearer came near. Then her mother found her in a rigid cataleptic trance and a male voice in broad American English spoke as Bert Relton who had been a famous band-leader during life on earth. He claimed to be her control and from that time phenomena occurred in trances and out of them especially when she called on Bert to perform. Evidently Bert was as keen to indulge in a bit of fun as Mrs. Shearer, and her brother Mr. R. Berger would challenge Bert to perform all sorts of feats. They would lock themselves in a room just the two of them and then ask Bert to remove any object from the room through locked doors and windows and place it somewhere in a conspicuous place. Afterwards when they opened the door they would find a vase or some ornament in some odd place on the staircase or kitchen. They would enter a room and lock a drawer with a new shirt inside then challenge Bert to do something with the shirt and a few minutes later when the drawer was unlocked the shirt was found tied full of knots.

One morning her brother left his bedroom for a bath but left his wrist-watch lying on his dressing table. When he returned the watch-strap was wound round and round the electric flex high up near the ceiling light. He had to stand on a stepladder to unloosen it.

During the same morning while sitting at breakfast with Mrs. Shearer in the diningroom a number of large wooden beads belonging to a broken necklace were lying on the other end of the table and while he was looking at them he passed some remark about the beads. The next moment they were jumping off the table on to the floor and back again on to the table. They put the beads on the sideboard and the two of them left the house for the flat where she normally lived. Some distance down the street her brother noticed to his consternation that some of the huge wooden beads were following them, rolling along the street and almost bouncing as they rolled on behind her. To avoid drawing the attention of passers-by he went back and picked up the beads.

Once during a seance a large jackal skin was lying on the floor near the door while in the middle of the room stood a table and high up near the ceiling was a light suspended from a short electric wire. To reach this light one had to stand on a chair placed on top of the table. The lights were extinguished for the seance but the witnesses stated that they could see each other dimly and would have noticed or heard anyone climbing on to the table with a chair; anyway when the trance was over and the lights were restored the jackal skin was wrapped around the wire and the light, actually tied round by its corners.

On an occasion of her birthday her mother and I visited her home and found three others there apart from her husband. He produced some sparkling red sweetish wine with which to toast his wife's health. Mrs. Shearer was sitting in an armchair facing me in her usual corner. Since her husband did not care for any of her phenomena and firmly believed that she was the chief agent, Mrs. Shearer never entered a trance-state in his presence. His attitude was derived from experience that at times these manifestations got out of hand and played havoc in his house and being a dour Scotsman such things did not appeal to him at all.

We finished our drink and Mr. Shearer came round to refill the goblet glasses. He naturally had to look into each glass to see where he was pouring the wine. If therefore there had been an object the size of an egg in a glass he would have seen it at once. Yet although he was walking around with the bottle to where his guests sat and carefully poured the wine neither he nor his guests made any remark about an egg in the wine glass. Mrs. Shearer was sitting in her corner and we again raised our glasses to her when as I lifted my glass to my lips I found something heavy and solid against my mouth.

I looked and there was a large hen's egg in my glass. All the others similarly found eggs in their glasses, except Mr. Shearer. His wife however claimed no knowledge of the whole affair and candidly she had not been near our wine glasses as far as anyone could recall. Besides if she had placed the eggs in the glasses after her husband had filled them with wine then by displacement of fluid the wine would have spilled over. If on the other hand she had put them in before he filled the glasses the second time then one of us must have seen a hen's egg at the bottom of a transparent wine goblet glass and Mr. Shearer looking in the direction in which he was pouring the wine should have seen the eggs.

This puzzle led to a lively discussion and Mr. Shearer accused his wife of playing one of her tricks. I was amused and wanted to know how it had happened for I knew Mrs. Shearer was not any good at sleight of hand. I had tested her for this ability on several occasions. Anyway during this discussion she appeared somewhat irritable and restless and she had a strange sort of mischievous expression. I who had seen this emotional pattern in the past preceding some poltergeist manifestations expected anything to happen. Her husband was still insisting that she had brought the eggs into the lounge and deposited them in our glasses when our attention was drawn to the other end of the room. Two eggs and tomatoes were squashed together as if slapped against the wall in one movement and in one spot high up near the ceiling of a room with high walls. The tomato juice and broken raw eggs were running straight down the wall. There was no scattering in the direction of throw as should have been the case if they had been thrown by Mrs. Shearer.

In any case there were other factors against a physical throw by her. The lounge was long and narrow and she was sitting in one corner while the eggs and tomatoes were squashed against the opposite wall about twenty-five feet away near the corner. If she had thrown these objects they could not all have landed together in the same spot. There would have been scattering and the fragments would have streaked in the direction of the throw whereas these were squashed together in a manner no visible individual could have done. These strange phenomena showed that at times Mrs. Shearer produced supernormal powers.

Once for instance during a trance there was a loud report and a platinum ring on her finger was split right through. On most occasions when I have observed these poltergeist phenomena they were associated with a mood condition. She herself described this state as a feeling of intense restlessness and a tremendous desire—almost an urge for something startling inexplicable and supranatural to happen. She often admitted that she did not visualize the nature of the manifestation but did look forward to the startled reaction of the audience; the surprised disturbed equilibrium in fact. Then at a certain stage this mood would pass and there would come a feeling of detachment with elation and exhilarating contemplation of what might occur. This mood of exaltation often preceded her best trance performances.

During her seances Bert Relton spoke very frequently and in a male voice with an American accent. Most of the great figures of the past communicated including poets, kings, statesmen and philosophers—Lord Alfred Tennyson, William Shakespeare, Moses of the Bible and so on. The wild poltergeist type of phenomena which marked the first years of her mediumship gradually changed as she entered a phase of ethical and spiritual addresses, emphasizing love and kindness towards our fellowmen. It was truly amazing to observe the multiplicity of qualities which she was capable of expressing. The range of her voice varied from deep bass tones to the most feminine and delicate qualities.

This was especially so when an angelic being known as Sympathea spoke. Her voice and speech exuded infinite gentleness and virtue. One heard in word and emotion a crystallization of tolerance and the acme of forgiveness and grace. One could not help but accept that Mrs. Shearer's feelings and ideas were illuminated by some inner light of the psyche. This voice cooed the words and there was a bell-like quality about them. They used to die away like the plucked muted notes of a stringed instrument.

Often however I noticed that other female spirits when emphasizing refinement of thought would cultivate the voice and tone of Sympathea. This gave the impression that Sympathea represented the purified ethereal pattern of trance communication. The medium was an elocutionist and at one time also an actress. Most of her characters spoke in Elizabethan English. Speech in Afrikaans however was not superior to the limited vocabulary and lack of practice in pronounciation which the medium displayed when she spoke Afrikaans out of trance. The communications as I have mentioned were almost entirely given to ideas of love, sympathy and kindness. Sympathea represented the quality of heavenly sympathy and her discourses were invariably beautiful. An example might convey the impression better than my description.

"I am this evening with thee from the centre. As ye seek so shall ye find. I have found consciousness within all of ye. I bestow my gifts of kindness of love and of comfort on you. Knowledge is love. Love is infinite. Knowledge is wisdom. Wisdom is ultimate. When your eyes are awakened to full consciousness nothing will seem immature. Your plane is the plane of appearances as we develop consciousness we are made to see and look upon the plane of appearances. We realize that on the plane you inhabit life-thought becomes one of appearance. When you arrive on this plane it is as clear as a crystal pool of water, for all appearances are but brief seasons within the life of man.

Let us not ask more of mortal man but to elevate his thoughts and those that seek and desire life's nobler influences will receive benefits. There is but one truth and it is veiled. We must not question the purpose of the Higher Most Celestial Mind. Power remains the combined association of all qualities within the human conception. Ye shall all feel the eternal when you have flung away all earth—only then can the power of contact with the highest be reached. Your search for knowledge is only the cause of the infinite celestial rays."

She would often speak in the same strain for an hour. One observes the emphasis on the question of faith without the word being mentioned. Now although these addresses usually consisted of poetical and abstract ideas which took the form of a series of disconnected pronouncements directed towards appreciation of spiritual grandeur they appeared as the personification of the medium's most reverential thoughts.

They gave no information about the nature of the spirit world but claimed an omnipotent quality in penetrating into the minds of the sitters and knowing their very thoughts. This exaltation must impress people not used to these prolonged discourses and such aesthetic appreciation. Thoughts like these would appeal to their finer natures. Yet there was nothing appertaining to knowledge about anything which could form a memory in one's mind even after one-and-a-half hours of continuous listening. It all disappeared in a delicate wreath of poetic phraseology; indeed wafted away by the slenderest threads of consciousness into nebulous regions.

What was of profound interest was the difference between speech and content and vocal ability during trance and that of Mrs. Shearer in her daily expression of thought. In my long association with her I never heard her express ideas in such phraseology nor make use of such novel forms of presentation. Even the magnificent array of platitudes had an atmosphere and origin, a range of association, meaning and symbolism of which the medium gave no evidence while out of trance. Nevertheless I could not help but feel that somehow there was a trance personality to which the subconscious mind of the medium made a substantial contribution.

She has never been known in my experience to entertain feelings of dislike or visible prejudice towards anyone. Her generous nature was always ready to wish goodwill on all who came in contact with her. She had for instance a firm faith that her spirit guide Bert Relton could perform miracles. It was apparent that by means of this wish, hope and desire she imagined almost in a child-like manner that things would happen for the happiness of others. Now I observed this same attitude of mind, this same imagined thought trend when other physical phenomena happened out of her trances. There was a decided mental endeavour to create effects by the power of wish; indeed a tendency to feel her way into people and things and to bring about her desires and wishes by this concentration of feeling. It was as if she wanted to manipulate things and bring about results by willing them to happen.

I became convinced that the physical trance phenomena and others occurred in consequence of this frame of mind. Even the eggs in our wine on the occasion of the birthday party as well as the eggs and tomatoes on the wall were the result of her desire to play a prank, to create excitement and to spring a surprise. She no doubt had similar intentions before entering a trance and so produced startling effects. Rudi Schneider moved objects and Anna Rasmussen willed them to move.

Mrs. Shearer claimed that she had no idea how these things happened but there was no doubt to my mind that the poltergeist type of phenomena were entirely dependent on her mood and wish. These were too numerous to mention but all of them left one impression—that there was a field of force which radiated from and surrounded the medium. The intensity of this field of force varied with her physical state and mood or the influence of people and the emotional atmosphere. The latter stimulated the need to act or indulge in some form of exhibitionism.

In my opinion this field of force could also respond to unknown laws of the physiology of the person. There were decidedly times when it was more extensive and more intense than at other times. It is my theory that when it reached a certain intensity it became susceptible to thought. At this intensity or potential it could be triggered to act on the astral or electronic constituents of material objects causing thereby forms of movement quite inexplicable by ordinary physical laws of action. The question arises whether only the medium's own thoughts could affect this field of force or whether the thoughts of discarnate beings could do the same?

It is of interest to note that the late General Smuts in his book "Holism and Evolution" mentioned that there was activity structuralised in bodies and things which extended beyond the object. This conception refers to the same idea as I have in mind but I assume this activity to be radiative and of an electromagnetic nature, capable of extending quite some distance beyond the confines of the physical body.

In the experiments with Rudi Schneider conducted by Dr.

Osty this emanation from the medium was capable of transmitting his rate of breathing to a galvanometer some distance away. It gives the impression of a sort of electromagnetic field of force which could make the galvanometer respond to its impulses; a force that could transmit invisibly the vital impulse of Schneider's respiratory rhythm. It is of interest to note in passing that although to my knowledge the late General Smuts in his philosophical speculations never investigated psychics yet his theory certainly finds support in the interpretation of these phenomena occurring in the presence of psychic persons.

My experience with Mrs. Shearer has led me to think that forms of energy of many different frequencies are radiated from the human organism. I have mentioned previously that we appear to be composed of many different wavebands of energy. I have for years entertained this conception which is so difficult to make explicit because of man's unknown power and because the idea is a product of intuition.

Will it ever become an objective biochemical fact or a mathematical proposition which could be proved by its logic? I think that among these many different wavebands of the human spectrum of energy there is one concerned with healing of disease or wounds and so on. This energy system might be of high potential in some people and medium or low in others. It might be that it could only indirectly be triggered by other wavebands of energy before its healing vibrations are released. Modern medicines such as the wide range of antibiotics, the sulphonomides and vitamines to mention only a few could by their chemical natures set up similar radiative healing powers. Maybe this is when the particles of physics are converted into waves. Radiations of this nature could attain a frequency rate of vibration which falls within the waveband of healing; so that these radiations from the biochemical and physical forms of energy could be stepped up to frequency rates whose potency could cure disease.

If we accept Sylvan Muldoon's theory that the astral body is a condenser and is charged with cosmic energy to be transmitted to the physical organism then perhaps we could consider the astral as the conductor of this higher frequency rate of vibration which results in healing. Such a process could thus be initiated from the astral psychological or from the biochemical side with its bioelectric energy transformation. It could perhaps also be potentiated from the psychic side of personality. Thought, prayer or perhaps discarnate thought processes could operate on this waveband in man. Such psychic forces could augment its power and intensity.

From the experience of my daughter which I am about to relate it does appear that this healing vibration can be conducted by any form of life. In fact that it is part of the spectrum of life and where life is there it could be stored. Maybe any living object could become charged with this power. The influence of discarnate thought taking part in the process of healing could operate by means of a higher frequency rate. Perhaps by these means there is a liberation of this power within the confines of the sick human organism.

It could on the other hand be that such discarnate or spiritual beings act as conductors from cosmic sources and so create a field of force which becomes confluent with the field of force of the mediumistic being. Hence healing vibrations could be transmitted in the same manner as the respiratory rate of Rudi Schneider was transmitted and received by an electrical apparatus. In the example of the little primula the healing power was absorbed by the life of the plant. This plant life was augmented and potentiated by this particular rate of vibration. It was stored and retained by the plant until conducted away by a human being in need. The evidence is that the plant discharged its power and died.

It happened one evening during a trance by Mrs. Shearer that a spirit who alleged he was Jesus spoke. He spoke in a most reverent, dignified quiet voice with long pauses and among other things mentioned his power of healing while on earth. This gave me the opportunity to discuss my theory which I have enumerated above. He said, "I shall give you evidence in support of your theory. Underneath the fringe of your chair you will find a small primula of flowers which I have taken from a pot-plant in the hall. (The door leading to the hall was locked.) You shall care for it and in time by guidance you will discover that theory has bloomed into fact." Thereafter he took his departure and the seance came to an end.

When the lights were turned on I found a tiny primula of flowers under my chair. The stem however was extremely short; in fact less than half-an-inch long. I secured it in my buttonhole with a little safety pin until I had decided what to do with it. I arrived home about midnight and placed my notes of the evening's proceedings in my study. While there my eyes fell on a tiny brown bottle about the size of my thumb, with a few small tablets in it. I removed the tablets, filled the little bottle with water and placed my primula in it. The tiny stem was about as long as the neck of the bottle was deep. Anyway it was submerged in water.

Every second day I put clean water in myself and no one was allowed to touch this bottle except when instructed by me. The flower was given to me some time in August. It kept on blooming and each morning tiny fresh blooms would open. This went on through August, September, October, November and during

December I went on holiday. I left instructions with Peter my trusted Rhodesian African male servant to attend to the little flower with great care and to change its water every second day. Peter had a great respect for this magic flower which, although kept in a tiny bottle continued blooming as if it were part of a huge plant. He remarked that the flower possessed great medicine. That remark was to say the least a little uncanny.

When we returned at the end of December the primula was still blooming, and most luxuriantly. So it went on throughout January and February and then my daughter, aged twelve, after repeated attacks of severe tonsillitis had to have her tonsils removed. After the operation she had a serious haemorrhage but when over the acute effects came home from the nursing home. The next morning I heard her crying bitterly because her throat was so painful and swollen that she could not swallow and she would not even attempt to do so. I examined her throat and found it an angry-looking swollen mass. Evidently there was still some infection and the resistance of the tissues was low.

I decided to call in the colleague who had performed the operation when suddenly a powerful impulse determined me to fetch the flower. The thought that came to me was that my daughter should hold the bottle with the flower in it in front of her open mouth and breathe in as if drawing into her throat the life of the flower. But she was not to breathe out over the flower—only in from it. She should continue to do so until the flower had wilted and until there was no more pain on swallowing. Having given her those instructions as they came to my mind I left for my consulting rooms in the city.

An hour-and-a-half later I thought of my daughter and the little flower. I telephoned my wife and was told, "Marlene is much better—the throat is no longer paining her. She has eaten a breakfast but your little flower has died." I went home at lunch-time, something which I seldom did and found to my amazement that my daughter was bright and that her throat looked much better. She could eat. The swelling had miraculously subsided. But my primula was dead. Although it was kept in the water in the bottle my daughter described how it wilted before her eyes. She could see the little petals droop and fall apart from each other. The little flower itself which had always remained upright in the bottle hung languidly and lifelessly over the neck of the little bottle.

I changed the water and kept it in its bottle hoping it would survive but it fell apart and its stem rotted. It was dead. The change in my daughter's throat was immediate. I have on several occasions told people this story of the long life of this tiny primula and its dramatic end when its life and its stored-up healing power was drawn out of it by the prayerful appeal of my daughter. Their reactions varied but were mostly superficial and tactful.

Here again were examples of people trying to explain away or reject in some way or other what their minds could not comprehend. It has been said that my daughter was cured by suggestion and faith because she knew the history of the primula. But one may ask—are these intelligent answers or explanations? Are the terms "suggestion" and "faith" not themselves in need of explanation? By what process do these functions of thought bring about a physical change? More reasonable is the idea of a certain rate of energy vibration which could be triggered by thought in the same manner as a field of force radiated by a person can be triggered into producing the invisible movement of objects.

Somehow thought remains the supreme frequency rate which manipulates these other wavebands provided their potentials are high enough. During the seven months that this little primula bloomed with a stem less than half-an-inch long more than its ordinary and usual life must have sustained it. Its stem would otherwise have rotted away within days. Secondly, this unique property of life which it revealed must be accepted as dating from the night it was given to me in a séance. The most rational explanation appears to be that the alleged spiritual communicant increased this rate of healing vibration in the medium.

In other words he knew of a technique to do so by means of thought. The medium's aura or field of force probably became highly charged with this type of energy of life. One can imagine how the little primula's tiny vital power acted as a conductor. In this capacity it stored up sufficient life-force to keep itself alive for seven months and thereafter it gave up its little life to heal an inflamed and swollen throat. Somehow life is the great host of all these mysterious powers which sometimes overflow their frontiers into our ordinary physical lives and so become manifestations of the paranormal.

CHAPTER III

POLTERGEIST MANIFESTATIONS

Bold startling headlines :

HAUNTED WOMAN IN HOSPITAL NOW, HUNDREDS WATCH GHOST HOUSE

were carried by the *Evening Post*, Port Elizabeth, giving the full name and address of a lady whom we shall call Mrs. A. for professional reasons. The press photographs showed the lady in hospital with scratch marks on her legs alleged to have been caused by the ghost.

The newspaper story which was authentic according to my investigations read : "A thirty-five-year old Port Elizabeth woman Mrs. A was taken to the Provincial Hospital last night after complaining that invisible, rough hands grabbed her by the throat and throttled her.

Earlier police had stood by helplessly while an invisible attacker seemed to hurl Mrs. A against a wall, rip her curtains to shreds and scratch her until blood flowed. At 3 a.m. today hundreds of people still thronged the street outside the house. Police arrested several men who tried to force their way into the house and then refused to leave. "We are exhausted. We cannot take any more Mrs. A's sister said today."

MURDERER HANGED

"Mrs. A spent today in hospital. Officials described her condition as satisfactory and she has not complained of being troubled further. No more unusual happenings were reported at the home where the rest of the family spent a quiet night. Mrs. A believes that the harrowing experiences of the past few days were caused by a curse. Her mother, Mrs. Anna Stevens was murdered at her home in October 1959. Mrs. A gave evidence at the trial which resulted in the hanging of a coloured man.

"After the trial stones mysteriously crashed through windows of her house. It was on Thursday morning that things started happening. Stones came flying into the house shattering windows and Mrs. A was hurled against a wall by what she described as 'strong invisible hands.'

"The police were called in but say they had to stand by helplessly while the invisible attacker sometimes threw her on the floor. Sergeant T. de Villiers of the Korsten Police went to the house on Thursday afternoon. He saw tables and chairs moving about with nobody near them. Curtains were ripped to shreds. Sergeant de Villiers helped to pin Mrs. A down on the bed when the invisible force seemed bent on hurling her against the wall. He said today 'I could feel some invisible force tugging violently at Mrs. A's shoulder. Her body was limp and she did not move. Once she was lifted bodily and flung on the floor in a limp bundle.' Constable B. J. Strydom of Korsten said that he immediately felt that there was something wrong when he entered Mrs. A's room. 'It was as if someone had thrown a cup of cold water down my back. I stood near the bed then walked to the door. Something took me by the shoulders and pulled me back towards the bed. I did not resist and found myself again standing at the bed.' Two policemen who helped to pin Mrs. A down were lifted by an invisible force and thrown on the floor. One had a bruise on his chest which he said came from the invisible attacker.

"The police fetched Mr. Charles Benjamin, a St. Helena man who claimed that he could drive away the evil spirit on Thursday afternoon. Shortly after he arrived Mrs. B fell asleep and everything was quiet. At midday yesterday the mysterious attacks on her resumed however. Mr. B, Mrs. A's brother-in-law described how she received the scratches on her arms and legs. 'She was sitting on a chair when she suddenly yelled, 'The thing has got me!' Then blood spurted from her arms and legs. There was no one near her and she did not scratch herself.' Last night with hundreds of people outside the house the family decided to take Mrs. A to hospital so she could have a good night's rest."

I read the above account in the newspaper and contacted the doctor who attended to Mrs. A and with his permission took over the case. I found a rather stout English-speaking woman who showed some scratches and repeated the story in the newspaper. She was genuinely frightened and seeking the protection of the nurses. She was given prolonged sleep and after a few days was removed to a private home because the hospital atmosphere was facilitating the development of childish dependence and the need for sympathy.

Careful investigation of Mrs. A's history revealed that she had had a most unfortunate childhood. At the age of three while toddling around in her granny's laundry she had swallowed caustic soda. Thereafter she was virtually a hospital patient until about fifteen years of age. She also suffered from attacks of loss of consciousness. She would feel dizzy and something would come up from her stomach and she would remember no more. After a while she would feel quite well again. Her father also suffered from similar attacks. She is still suffering from these attacks although they are controlled by the necessary medication.

To return to her childhood years. Because of her repeated and prolonged stay in hospital she had very little schooling. She was very dependent on the love and sympathy of the family and would be easily upset if harshly treated. She worked in a factory and did very well at her job in spite of the fact that attacks of loss of consciousness occurred during her work. When these attacks became more frequent at the age of eighteen years she became blind. According to the doctor who attended her at that time this was an hysterical blindness.

She was taken by her parents accompanied by her fiance (who fell in love with her during her blind period) to see an Xosa witch-doctor somewhere near Seymour. He told them that she had been bewitched by a man who had been rejected by her sister and who had buried some medicines near the doorstep. Unfortunately Mrs. A instead of her sister had stood on this medicine and so she had become afflicted with blindness. He gave her several bottles of medicines and herbs to drink. She was cured after six months. The evil powers of witchcraft were driven away.

Mrs. A staunchly believes that this is so, even today. She had several children and apart from the queer attacks of loss of consciousness carried on fairly contentedly in spite of domestic and financial problems. After her mother had been murdered coloured men came to her house and threatened her that they would kidnap her little daughter if her evidence convicted their friends. Stones were thrown at the house but these were apparently thrown by hooligans to intimidate her. She firmly believed in spite of the physical evidence of people who were seen that the forces of witchcraft would be turned loose again and cause something terrible to happen to her, maybe she would become blind again.

Then in 1961 she had members of her family staying with her and there were financial worries and lack of food. She had no money for cigarettes and also had a great deal of pain in her back and side. While in this depressed and miserable state of mind someone threw a stone through the window but the culprit was actually seen running away. So that this stone, the first at that time was not from an invisible or poltergeist source. Mrs. A panicked, became excited and believed firmly that ghostly forces were at work.

Now living in the home and present at this time was her sister's daughter aged sixteen years who also had emotional difficulties. It was actually this girl who saw a flower-pot full of earth with a pot-plant slide along the passage to the front door from its stand. Mrs. A saw this flower-pot passing her bedroom door and lost complete control of herself. At this stage stones began to fall as if coming from nowhere. Kitchen utensils were pulled off the shelves by invisible means. A milk bottle did a somersault in full view of them and in the immediate presence of the girl of sixteen. A heavy kitchen table was lifted clean off the floor and moved about five feet away. The rest of the happenings with police witnesses were as described by the newspaper report.

Once Mrs. A. came under psychiatric observation with psychotherapy she settled down. Her physical condition was investigated and it was found that she had stones in a kidney; this necessitated the removal of the kidney. Her losses of consciousness were diagnosed, treated and controlled. Mrs. A. is still under continuous treatment for this disturbance of brain rhythm. At present she is well and no more poltergeist phenomena have occurred.

She described how the ghost catcher made a little effigy of a little black man and stuck pins into its body in order to kill the ghost. It was quite apparent that these poltergeist phenomena ceased once a serious attempt was made to help Mrs. A. to form a rational conception of the happenings. After the ghost catcher had performed his rites the poltergeist came back with renewed vigour but disappeared dramatically the moment the psychological security of the hospital assuaged the mind. Now what is the explanation of all these strange obstreperous and even violent forces which operated in a manner of intelligent direction in the home of Mrs. A.?

We have seen that her emotional make-up and personality pattern was prone to severe hysteria. Her unfortunate childhood, cultural background and losses of consciousness all produced a dependence and inner insecurity which left a poorly integrated personality. She grew up with a firm belief in witchcraft and a limited rational resistance to these strange but primitive ideas. With this poor emotional integration and constitutional anomalies as well there emerged a personality with a vivid and dramatic imagination. She became obsessed with the idea of unseen persecution and the possible kidnapping of her child. For months prior to the poltergeist appearance she was afraid to stay in the house alone during the day. She visited the neighbours and relatives until the children came home from school. She was tense, anxious and frightened of the unknown.

Now one must assume that she probably also had the capacity to build up a mediumistic field of force similar to Mrs. Shearer, Anna Rasmussen and Rudi Schneider to mention only these few. But I am of the opinion that the sister's daughter of sixteen was also a source for generating and radiating this energy system or field of force. A combination of these psychic power units directed by a firm belief in malign and depraved spirits could have caused the poltergeist phenomena. In addition there was the thought that the murderer who had been hanged would revenge himself. The evidence points to it that this field of force is directed by ideas, patterns of thought and impulses of mind.

I have suggested that its possible mode of action is on the electronic constituents of the object to be moved. In other words that it manipulates an energy system of a lower frequency rate to produce physical results. If my hypothesis is accepted that the astral body is the real personality then one must conclude that any will to action must proceed from the astral consciousness and the astral substance to a lower frequency forming the ectoplasmic in materialized manifestations. At a lower level one will have to postulate a slower rate of vibration of energy forming the field of force which produces physical action.

The picture is one of gradations of energy systems of different frequency rates from the astral to the neuromuscular. Quite a complex pattern of different energy levels with an almost corresponding picture in the physical organization of the central nervous system. Hence mind obsessed with the emotional power of belief, finding such a field of force at its disposal could perhaps produce some extraordinary phenomena. Her own subconscious ideas might attack Mrs. A. and so fulfill her expectations and fears. But could such a rational explanation be considered to account for all cases of poltergeist hauntings and disturbances? It cannot be denied that however imbecilic the pattern of ghostly behaviour might be it is not a blind force but a power with intelligent design and purpose. So that we must associate it with mind.

Now need it always be the minds of living people, in fact the victims of the phenomena? or could these disturbances also be produced by the minds of discarnate beings? It is commonly believed, and Outa Jantjes for instance who was evidently clairvoyant, insisted that there were those who did not seem to know they were really dead—they kept on wanting to do the things which they had done during life, for he had often seen them long before dawn helping to inspan the mules for ploughing. All this might have been the product of his imagination, but these experiences are accepted by people not given to phantasy. There are those who believe that there are beings in astral form whose minds are not different from depraved earthly behaviour.

Sylvan Muldoon describes an astral attack by one of these discarnate beings on the densest levels of the astral plane. If therefore mind can survive with these propensities, what should prevent it from influencing a mediumistic field of force or aura and then proceed to execute by means of this power its obsessive or aggressive ideas? Logically there appears to be no reason if we accept the survival of mind to deny it the ability to act on this field of force.

Controlled experiments have shown that some such process cannot be excluded as an explanation. I do not imply that Mrs. A. was attacked by the vengeful ideas of the murderer—her own ideas could have produced the effects. To my way of thinking it is wise to bear in mind that discarnate entities enslaved by earthly motives and ideas could perhaps gain control of this field of force which is radiated from one's physical being. With this hypothesis in mind one should study each haunt or poltergeist manifestation on its merits.

The term "Poltergeist" is derived from the German—polter to rattle, make a noise and generally behave boisterously and geist means simply spirit. So that it signifies a noisy, rattling racketing spirit. These outstanding characteristics have been the same wherever they have appeared in our world. Some of the chief components are banging of doors, falling crockery, opening doors, moving objects, heavy footsteps, blows or raps on floor, under beds and furniture, and sometimes disappearance of objects from locked rooms as in the case of Mrs. Shearer. Anyway the pattern seems to be motivated by a mind that wants to draw attention to itself quite apart from some apparent exhibitionistic trends.

The action-results tend to convey some idea of the level of intelligence employed and this corresponds to something rather naive and childish or even imbecilic. On the whole it seems so stereotyped as if the intelligence of a certain level has a certain pattern of expression to convey some need or to give vent to some aggression or to startle, upset and frighten people with the motives of a practical joker. Someone once asked whether poltergeist manifestations are not caused by earthbound circus clowns? Anyway the clown pattern of behaviour seems often to fit the poltergeist most admirably.

It is amazing to perceive the amount of magical nonsense which our lower strata of society believe. Ignorance of psychic matters lay these poor people open to all sorts of practitioners who farm on these pastures of unbounded credulity. "The Evening Post" Port Elizabeth carried the following headlines on another occasion :

BLACK MAGIC SPELLS AID THE ACE GHOST SLAYER.

"A ghost in the house? Mr. Charles Benjamin, a Port Elizabeth "ghost catcher" says you can get rid of it if you have some spipeta, rooiliefmaak, angelier and kershout. He says all these ingredients must be burned together, ground into a fine grey-black powder and then strewn inside the haunted house. Mr. Benjamin added another "dead ghost" to his list recently when he was called to rid a house in Despatch of a ghost that was alleged to have throttled a woman. The woman Mrs. M. E. de Jager said after Mr. Benjamin's visit "The depressed feeling and dizziness in my head are gone. We told Mr. Benjamin to kill the ghost." She said Mr. Benjamin lured the ghost into a car and then took it away.

"Recently the police fetched Mr. Benjamin and took him to a haunted house in Haupt Street Port Elizabeth. A woman said a ghost pricked her with a needle and assaulted her."

The newspaper continued :—

"According to Mr. Benjamin catching ghosts is an exhausting business. 'I was nearly dead after disposing of the ghost in Haupt Street. It was a very exhausting business.' The true story about Mrs. A is considerably different."

The reporter went on to say :—

"When I visited Mr. Benjamin's house at Veerplaats there were several white women and coloured men waiting in the dimly lit sittingroom to see Mr. Benjamin. In his room behind a sliding door were a farmer and his wife from George. They had come all the way to see Mr. Benjamin in the hope that he could cure their daughter whose legs were swollen. The mother said she believed someone had cast an evil spell over her daughter. On the table in the room stood a bottle filled with herbs and a pale foaming liquid. Mr. Benjamin mysteriously tucked a paper with something scribbled on it into his vest pocket. 'I'll tell you a secret,' he whispered. 'Pepper, white chalk and salt—and prayer—is a strong medicine.'

"He showed me photographs of scores of white women and men who had come to see him, some from as far as Johannesburg. Most wanted Mr. Benjamin to bring loved ones back to them. Many were men who had been deserted by their wives. In a drawer Mr. Benjamin keeps pieces of clothing of all the people whom he is to bring back. A pair of pants for instance was brought to him by a Port Elizabeth woman who said her husband had kicked her out of the house. 'Could Mr. Benjamin make him love her again?' "

I have quoted sufficiently from this press interview with a "ghost catcher" who also specialises in the magic of love potions to reveal the strata of belief and primitive mentality which share religion and technological benefits with all of us. This hidden subjective world of man in which he is so often a small child in his beliefs has been untouched by education and religion. Education is not concerned with psychic phenomena but evidently also not with the data of human personality that could help man to emancipate himself by his efforts of mind from the magical and infantile strata of his emotional thinking.

Another press report described how a soup tureen full of soup was taken from the table and emptied on the floor, also coffee was poured on the floor by invisible means as well as boiling water. Burning sticks of wood and red-hot coals were plucked by invisible hands from the fire and thrown on the floor. Brown spittles of tobacco juice fell on the shoulders of the people in the house. All this had been happening at the time of the report for sixteen days in the home of Mr. F. R. Nel of Amherst on the other side of the Katberg.

Mr. Nel who is eighty-two said "his nerves were done from all this witchcraft and haunting." It is said that the Amherst ghost also spoke to the people of the house. He had nevertheless broken a number of things and would grab cups and saucers and smash them against other objects. The family had often to be careful to avoid being hit by these flying bits of crockery.

Mrs. J. S. C. Nel of Kleinbegin near Queenstown, a daughter-in-law of Mr. Nel of Amherst said that when a cup of coffee is placed on a table it is immediately snatched away and thrown on the floor. A seventeen-year-old girl was burnt on the arm by the ghost. A Swahili man said that the ghost was brought by someone working in the house. The ghost himself has said that he is carrying out the wishes of a native woman known as Mompsi who wants to take revenge on Mr. Nel senior. The ghost does not disturb them during the day, only at night.

It is of importance to note that the newspaper report only deals with the dramatic news value and is silent on the number of people in the house, the number of servants and their ages. The possibility of a mediumistic personality—black or white in the house is not considered. The newspaper hence does not attempt to throw any light but merely repeats the system of belief.

An enlightened press for instance which is not prepared merely to be a mouthpiece of the dramatic and the startling but is also prepared to bring new ideas to bear on these problems could be extremely helpful in research of this nature. One must accept provisionally that as was the case with Mrs. A there was some person in the house who hence radiated a field of force or aura of such intensity that certain thoughts could perform acts of annoyance or express the vengefulness of someone with a grievance. These ideas in the mind of a servant who has such an intense field of force could perhaps be augmented from physical as well as discarnate sources.

Further examples might illustrate aspects to show whether the discarnate hypothesis is valid. Mr. Sadie furnished me with the following investigation by himself and a Mr. Vorster in March 1954 at Hurst Hill, Johannesburg. Mrs. Nieuwoudt the lady of the house said that they had lived there for two years and all was peaceful until March 1954 when stones rained on the roof and later window panes were smashed. At times lumps of coal were thrown, and Mrs. Nieuwoudt observed that the lump of coal would travel in a half-circle before it landed. This shows that it was not thrown by physical means but was transported by some medium of energy which could change the course of its transportation.

On occasions all the windows were shut and yet the stones seemed to come in at the windows, at least they dropped as if coming in at the windows—but not a single window pane was broken. The next day the stones would come crashing through the window panes again. Thirty-one window panes were broken and the police were constantly on guard but could not catch any culprit. Mr. Sadie found the house in chaos; lumps of coal and stones all over the house, even in the bathroom and many window panes were smashed. These were broken almost in the presence of the police on duty. The Captain of the police said that no one could have thrown those stones from the outside.

Mr. Sadie as an experienced investigator discovered that Mrs. Nieuwoudt had a little native servant aged twelve years and that the stones seemed to have been drawn towards her presence. The Nieuwoudts had brought this girl from the farm to Johannesburg and allowed her to sleep in the house and not in the servant's room because of her youth and nervousness. They observed that she had been hit several times by the stones. The stone throwing took place between nine and ten in the morning and three to four o'clock in the afternoon. Sometimes however it continued into the night but not as a rule. Whenever strangers or visitors came to the house the phenomena usually ceased immediately.

When the police first arrived the manifestations disappeared while they were there but after a few days somehow lost respect for the uniform and the stones would fall whenever a policeman had his attention diverted. Mr. Sadie suggested that the little native girl could be the source of action, and explained how these phenomena required a medium. It was not necessary for her to be conscious of the process. He even offered to take the girl to his home and keep her under observation for a few days. But Mrs. Nieuwoudt would not hear of this since the girl had been entrusted to them by her parents; besides she refused to accept the possibility that the servant girl could be an unconscious medium. They were convinced that the whole thing was the work of witchcraft and consulted a person versed in the power of witchcraft.

He burned all sorts of concoctions and the phenomena ceased immediately. Even Mr. Sadie was temporarily impressed. The Nieuwoudts sold their house in Hurst Hill and left for Van Wyksrust taking their little servant girl with them. They however were hardly settled in their new home when the same stone throwing and poltergeist phenomena started with renewed vigour. This case has certain interesting features which suggest that indirect emotional effects on the subconscious, such as fear and belief in the potency of witchcraft remedies could for a time inhibit or prevent this pattern of power expression.

The phenomena ceased when strangers or visitors came to the house. This also happened while the police had a certain amount of awe-inspiring effect on the little servant girl, but once she saw them day after day and became used to the idea, the stone throwing would happen stealthily as if it were something that had to be done and could not be restrained. It almost seemed to avoid being caught by the law. The same emotional restraining effect took place when the servant saw the rigmarole of ludicrous magical rites performed in which her mistress and master evidently believed.

These are to my mind subconscious inhibitions working through conditioned mental mechanisms and perhaps closely related to the energy system which causes this electromagnetic field of force or aura. Mrs. Nieuwoudt herself might have been an unconscious medium and so augmented this pattern of expression of a primitive and infantile destructive nature coming from the servant. No one really inquired as to whether this little girl was happy so far away from her family and associates. There is often longing, nostalgia or subdued unhappiness in these cases. The fact that the phenomena restarted at Van Wyksrust was proof in itself that the fear which the girl had of the anti-witchcraft remedies did not apply to the new home for the rites were not performed there and so the whole business started afresh.

An unhappy and lonely mood-state, in spite of the kindness of the Nieuwoudts could be considered as a reasonable motivation for poltergeist expression by one of this girl's culture and mental development. Hence subconscious urges, yearnings or intense emotional stress could very well overflow into this natural field of force of the personality and start phenomena but the effects will depend on the strength of the field of force. If such a person is mediumistic or is temporarily passing through a phase, when these various natures of the personality or wavebands of energy are for bioelectric or hormonic reasons poorly integrated then these expressions of a poltergeist nature could occur.

I know of two ladies who at fourteen and sixteen years of age or thereabouts found themselves possessed by urges of restlessness or desires for some form of physical expression and excitement and to their amazement objects fell about the place by mysterious means. These episodes were short-lived and happened only on one day and never recurred again but these ladies had a decided psychic temperament and were clairvoyant. Where however the attacks by the poltergeist are not only destructive and noisy in a three-year old manner, but became vicious, aggressive and assaultive, and the mediumistic person is a member of the family who suffers, but is not an unhappy member of that family then one should consider the possibility of a discarnate entity being implicated.

An astral being with earth life inclinations might take possession of such a mediumistic field of force or aura and if it has at its command power for the production of physical effects, it could express an urge which its earthbound state appears to facilitate. The following case taken from Mr. Sadie's collection will illustrate the above point of view.

In July 1957 an African man complained to the police at Nigel that there was a "thing" in his house causing chaos and running wild. Constables C. la Grange and C. L. van Tonder went to the farm Bultfontein two miles from Nigel to investigate the matter of the complaint. When they entered the African's house Constable la Grange was hit over the head with a broom while no one was anywhere near him. Constable van Tonder and a newspaper reporter and a photographer herded the members of the family into one room and shut the doors which were well secured. Ten minutes later the bedding was lying outside the house on the ground and in one room in which there was no one a mattress had caught fire.

The constables reported to their seniors and so Sergeant Deysel went to conduct an investigation, and he also was confronted by things being thrown about by invisible means. After this the Station Commander Head Constable H. C. Erasmus together with the Public Prosecutor Mr. J. Havenga and a Mr. C. F. Pretorius a miller, went to see what light they could throw on the ghostly phenomena.

When they arrived there was a fair crowd of curious people. The Head Constable again herded the family including a daughter of fourteen into one room and he placed a cordon of police and other white spectators around the house. They sat and waited for something to happen. A man sitting next to the Head Constable gave it as his opinion that the only remedy was to take a sjambok and hit the air in all directions. He was still busy describing what should be done when some invisible being hit him a blow which staggered him. He immediately accused the Head Constable who denied all knowledge or intention of such a deed.

After this blow was struck things began to move in earnest. Mr. Havenga was hit against the head with a spoonful of porridge and the miller Mr. Pretorius was hit against the head with a plate full of porridge. Head Constable Erasmus was amused at this and remarked to the miller that the ghost did not care for his flour. Hardly had the words left him when some invisible being hit him five blows on the head. A tray on a table began to dance and a bicycle in a corner fell over but its back wheel was spinning at speed. In another room a cupboard with crockery, and a fairly heavy one was lifted off its stand and placed in a leaning position against the wall.

Another eye-witness Mr. Pat Smith of Nigel was sitting on his haunches puffing at his pipe when the pipe was jerked out of his mouth and later found in a shoe under a bed. Then a chair came sailing through the room and hit the mirror of a wardrobe and smashed it. A bottle came towards the Head Constable, brushed against his head and then smashed itself against the wall. The family of the house hardly ever had any sleep. I do not know how it all ended, but Mr. Sadie mentioned that Professor M. Valkhoff, the Chairman of the South African Association for Psychic Research said in a press statement that he suspected the fourteen-year old girl who lived in the house as the cause of the phenomena.

Again we do not know the girl's emotional relationship with the family, especially whether she had a grievance or was unhappy. The sustained aggressive, vindictive and assaultive behaviour cannot be attributed to someone who is a happy member of a family. One is then driven to the possible explanation that this fourteen-year old girl was not only mediumistic but that her aura of field of force was invaded by an earthbound astral inhabitant who was working off his earthly aggressive trends, anger or paranoid motivations in this manner. The main principle to follow in all such cases of poltergeist manifestations is to look for the mediumistic person and thereafter to investigate the psychological state of such a person.

It might be advisable where possible to remove such a person from the environment during psychotherapeutic investigation and treatment. I am in possession of hundreds of letters referring to the poltergeist type of haunt. These indicate that the phenomena are quite common. But one gains the impression that they all seem to occur most frequently on a certain cultural level of society, especially among the poorer classes—white, coloured and African. It is highly suggestive that the mental world of those people play a dominant role. Their traditional beliefs, superstitions and infantile magical explanations, as well as the emotional make-up of the personalities are all factors which have a hand in shaping the pattern of the phenomena.

In a way it does resemble a mental process which is known in medical psychology as catharsis. This term literally means "purging." It affords an opportunity of working off natural impulses which were once important and which could not be gratified by natural means. It could also be a process of freeing repressed emotions as in the case of the unhappy Grietje. One could call this a form of poltergeistic abreaction. Aristotle applied this term to a purging of fear or anger by seeing the representation of these on the stage in tragedy. These psychological mechanisms might be employed by earthbound astral beings to play off their stressful emotions through channels provided by the aura of a mediumistic personality.

The following report appeared in a newspaper : "Mr. and Mrs. W. van Niekerk of "The Valley" in Elands River Valley have suffered losses amounting to a few hundred rand as a result of a poltergeist. Curtains were torn from the windows, pieces of furniture were knocked about and broken and clothes were torn from Mr. van Niekerk's body. The foam-rubber cushions were cut into pieces. Several large photographs which hung high up on the walls disappeared before their eyes and were later found behind a hill broken to smithereens. Pots and pans were hammered and ruined. Windows were smashed and sheets were cut into shreds while the couple were asleep in bed. Mr. van Niekerk's suspicions fell on a native woman on the farm and he ordered her away. They then went for a short holiday and on their return all manifestations had ceased. The woman had left the farm."

Here the farmer acted intelligently and suspected some person as being the source of this strange power. These poltergeist manifestations are understood among Afrikaners and Cape coloured as "goelery." This is a Malay-Afrikaans term and seems to signify the magic power by means of which an ordinary physically alive personality can be made invisible for the purpose of carrying out his nefarious deeds. It is believed that this power of witchcraft could be employed to turn a servant into a baboon, an ape or a huge dog. Thereafter the inmates of a home are frightened and harrassed by these pseudo-creatures.

There are South African white people of the poorer classes, Coloureds and Malays, who firmly believe in the existence of a magical power in the universe which can be manipulated by certain rites and so transform people or make them invisible. These people are unable to accept a mediumistic explanation such as I have advanced but they will readily accept the most primitive beliefs of witchcraft. It is this system of belief in "goelery" which makes it possible for the most absurd methods of ghost catchers to be believed and consulted such as the gentleman who lured a ghost from a house into a motor car and then drove it away. On another occasion he caught one and put it in a bottle and then corked the bottle so that it could not escape. The ghost was killed in this manner.

This vast strata of fantastic ignorance forms the mental material on which the charlatans who profess to wield magic make their living. The ancient beliefs and superstitions of witchcraft still have thousands of minds enslaved as a result of emotional immaturity and wishful thinking. During my field work among the Tembu people I found it a common belief that certain mythical creatures such as the Tikoloshe, the Impundulu and the Momlambo could change themselves into other beings and so deceive man while on their sinister missions.

These beliefs are part of the substance of witchcraft among the people. But I often wondered whether the isanuses actually believed in these powers of transformation. Because the true isanuse is a psychic person with good extrasensory perceptive faculties. In my association and friendship with Solomon Daba the amazing psychic witchdoctor I was given the impression that some witchdoctors are capable of producing thoughtforms which others could see.

It is a question of course whether these thoughtforms or phantasms could be made to haunt a person or act in the manner of poltergeists. Could such a thoughtform for instance take control of the field of force or aura of a psychic personality, and so perform a series of boisterous destructive and aggressive actions as a form of revenge, or for some other ulterior motive? The mechanism of "goelery" if at all possible could only take place by such means. Solomon Daba told me he could do this. I wondered however whether he was not merely boasting.

There is a modicum of support for this conception in the amazing experiences and achievements of Madam Alexandra David Neel which she clearly set out in her book "With Mystics and Magicians in Tibet." Madam Neel lectured in scientific circles in Paris on her return and also at the famous University of Sorbonne. She described how she learned to create a thoughtform companion who ultimately became a nuisance and was physically visible to her. In the end it took her three months to rid herself of this undesirable creature of her own creation.

This then was a well-known practice of the hermits of Tibet but I should say that the substantiality of the thought was due to the existence of a field of force. Thought had to have another medium which it could mould. This reminds one of the well-known telepathic phantasms of the living which have been seen without death or disaster. In how far the astral dimensionality has anything to do with these manifestations is difficult to say but I do believe that the substantial appearance of the thought form is dependent on a field of force radiated from a personality. The question remains open whether a projected thoughtform could account for what is known in South Africa as "goelery."

The following is said to be an authentic account of a ghost in a house in Oudtshoorn. It was sent to me by a person in a responsible position in the State Service and he believed it. In an old double storey house lived some tenants who were told to leave because the owner wanted to take occupation herself. It took a great deal of time and trouble as well as bad friendship to remove the tenants. Then as soon as the owner went to live there footsteps were heard at night. The bed on which she and her seven-year-old son slept was lifted clean off the floor and the floor-boards creaked during the night as if a heavy person were walking over them. Stones also rained on the roof but no one was seen throwing them. The police were sent for but they could not find any culprit. Then one day a mason came looking for work and she told him about this terrible noise and ghostly deeds. He said that she should have the old stove taken out as he considered the trouble was behind the stove.

She agreed and the mason obtained the job of removing the old stove which was bricked in and he put a new one in its place. Behind the old stove they found a piece of white wood, about two feet long. They burned this some distance from the house and from that time there were no more disturbances. I mention this account to illustrate the superstitious and traditional belief system which makes such utterly irrational and preposterous if not asinine thinking possible.

The unemployed mason makes a suggestion which provides him with a job. They find a piece of wood with all the magic powers for causing stones to fall and creating heavy footsteps on the creaking floors. The mason builds in a new stove and all is well. One does not know who the other poeple in the house were, who the servants were or whether for a time the lady herself was not an unconscious medium. She could have radiated the power in which ideas of persecution by erstwhile tenants precipitated the manifestations.

It does appear that when a piece of wood was conveniently found by the mason who wanted a job, her system of belief facilitated the conviction that all was over and the phenomena came to an end. It was not what was consciously thought but what was going on in a deeper level of consciousness.

I recently opened a newspaper to read in bold black headlines :

TIKOLOSHE (U.S. MODEL) ON A SPREE

The report came from Indianapolis where the police were baffled by crystal and china flying through the air. The house owner, Mrs. Renata Beck aged thirty-two years told of three days and two nights of frightening experiences. She and her mother watched cups, saucers, lamps, ashtrays and figurines crash to the floors or shatter against walls. She scoffed at suggestions that a poltergeist was responsible.

One finds in most of these reports that what complies with news value is often an extraction of dramatic elements, with suggestions leaning towards the basic witchcraft and superstition of common man, even to the extent of introducing a U.S. model of the African Tikoloshe. These mass media of communication employ an emotional medium which resembles the poltergeist in so far as that it at least must be startling.

A colleague in Cape Town sent me an account of a haunt in his surgery. He used to have a flat towards the rear of the building for two years, now he lives away and the maid sleeps in the back room. After he had fallen asleep while staying there he was awakened by some heavy footsteps, tramping around in his surgery, pulling out drawers and generally behaving like someone looking for something. There was even noisy rattling of his medicine bottles as if someone was imitating dispensing in a ludicrous manner.

He did not think these sounds paranormal but was annoyed at his disturbed sleep. But each and every maid complained of this nightly visitor. In the last few years the ghost imitated the typewriter being used. The present maid saw an apparition one night of a native girl of about fourteen coming into her room and sitting on her bed. The maid questioned her and the girl replied that she came from Kimberley and was looking for a friend.

On six occasions he had clerics to visit the place to say prayers with the object of exorcising the ghost over a ten-year period. But during the last nine months the noises have stopped, and my colleague no longer lives there. Somewhere in that house was an unconscious medium. The maid for instance who saw the apparition was probably psychic, and so provided the field of force whereby these physical effects such as sounds of dispensing and typing were produced.

Although Muldoon found that his astral body could on occasions develop the power to move physical objects, it must be remembered that Muldoon was not dead, and that he could draw on the neuric force or lower frequency rates of radiative energy. I think this dimensionality normally mediates the energy between mind and body and so leads to physical action. Hence one can accept as a general principle that a ghost must have an audience and it must have a source of power, and the latter is usually provided by living physical beings.

Mr. Sadie provided me with an interesting case which he called "The Ghost of Melville." These strange happenings took place in the home of Constable J. C. Burger of 82 Fifth Avenue Melville. While Mrs. Burger and three small children were home in the afternoon they heard a noise in some of the back rooms. It sounded as if someone were pushing the furniture about. Constable Burger arrived home at that moment, and searched his home from end to end but could not find anything responsible for the noise.

Then for a few days nothing happened, all was quiet and peaceful. Then suddenly one Friday the devil was let loose. During that night they heard all sorts of sounds and on the Saturday morning they found clothes scattered all over the house in the greatest disorder. A few garments were hanging from the trellis outside a bedroom window but nothing was missing. Constable Burger's brother who lived with them was listening with Mrs. Burger to the radio at about 9 p.m. when they heard a terrific noise in a back room. They rushed to the room and found that a window which had been latched was standing wide open and garments were hanging from the trellis outside as before.

Even after the constable had arrived home exactly the same thing happened, and no matter how they searched no valid cause was found. The whole of Saturday and that night were peaceful. But when they woke on the Sunday morning they found the house in a state of chaos. Garments were scattered all over the place, taken form wardrobes and chests of drawers. Two latched windows were wide open. Tins with plants growing in them had been removed from the garden and placed all over the kitchen and a lamp was found in a plant-pot at the back door.

Constable Burger's uniform had been taken from its usual place in the bedroom and hung up in a window of the lounge. The window was open but nothing was missing. While the family were having their breakfast after order had been restored a dish of breakfast food disappeared from under their noses off the table. By this time they were so upset that they 'phoned the police and went to the lounge to await them. While going along the passage Mrs. Burger felt someone jerking at the belt of her dress, but they saw no one. They were no sooner in the lounge however when someone invisible plucked the belt from her waist before their eyes and tied it round her neck.

The two men were completely taken by surprise to behold before their eyes how an invisible being wound the belt round her neck into a knot, and started to strangle her, all within split seconds. Only when she began to suffocate from strangulation did they jump at her and tear the belt from her neck. The next day the mark cf the belt was still red around her neck.

The police searched thoroughly but could not find a clue. By this time Constable Burger was almost desperate and he decided to nail a warning notice to the door which read as follows : "Leave my property in peace. Do not disturb it in any way. There is someone who is stronger than you. Be careful and be warned. Write down your name and address please." The ghost however showed his contempt of the police to such an extent that they found the warning notice on the ground smeared with human excreta. The front door was locked as usual, and no other disturbances took place that night except the unpleasant and filthy ghostly attention to the warning notice.

Then the next morning at about 8 o'clock Mrs. Burger found the pantry window broken with mud streaks all over shelves and broken glass scattered all over the house and outside as well. They found the wires leading to the radio set cut, and while Mrs. Burger was preparing lunch a whole cabbage just disappeared. But later the heart of the cabbage only was found under a sofa.

Then for the following three months all was quiet, nothing out of the ordinary happened. But for no known reason all of a sudden potatoes started flying all over the place as if they were just thrown or dropped. Money just fell from the pockets of people and tinkled on the floor. At this time Constable Burger's father- and mother-in-law, Mr. and Mrs. J. J. Olivier from South-West Africa came for a visit. While mother and daughter were peeling potatoes in the kitchen all the potatoes just vanished from the table.

While this was happening Mr. Olivier was standing next to a little bed of one of the children in their bedroom when he shouted that potatoes were raining on the bed, and one was ultimately found between the mattress and the springs. After this episodic display or impulsive exhibition four months elapsed in peace.

Now came an interesting turn of events which indicated that either the constable or his wife were the source of attraction or provided the power for these poltergeist phenomena. They went on a holiday to Kuruman and although all was quiet while they were at home, things began to happen once they were at

Kuruman. They were not long there on the farm when furniture was shoved about, shoes were thrown all over the place, coffee and sugar disappeared from the table and a lamp was lit in broad daylight; spoons and forks were seen falling in the house for no visible reason at all and bedding was hidden in all sorts of odd places.

Then somewhere during November 1954 after their vacation in Kuruman, Mrs. Burger heard the front door open and shut. A little later she heard her baby of ten months crying. She had left the baby in his cot in her bedroom but when she got there the baby was gone, and she found her crying baby in the children's bedroom. By three o'clock that afternoon the baby had disappeared. They could not find him anywhere. The search went on everywhere until ultimately there remained only one locked wardrobe, and when they unlocked this there was the ten-month old baby inside.

A few nights later while the family was asleep the ghost showed he had a sense of humour. He took the tunic of Constable Burger's uniform, his shoes and his helmet, and with the help of a few pillows and cushions he made a realistic police doll and placed it on a chair in the lounge. He however threw the other cushions on the floor and pushed the "pram" in the place where a little table with flowers stood and placed the table in the doorway.

The next day Mrs. Burger's wrist-watch disappeared and was later found in her powder box. Also while the constable was dressing for duty his cap was lying nearby when suddenly it was gone, and after quite a search was found on top of some blankets in the children's room.

Mr. Sadie described his personal investigations of this case especially one evening when in his presence the baby was put in his cot in the parents' bedroom. The other two children of three and two slept in their own room. Mr. Sadie personally shut the bedroom door. When after some time they entered the bedroom again, the baby was not in his cot but was sitting fast asleep right on top of a high wardrobe. There he sat as if a pair of invisible hands were holding him erect in his sleep. Mr. Burger's brother-in-law leapt forward to grab the baby, because his position and attitude without any visible support looked so precarious, but as he touched the child he fell limply forward into his hands in a relaxed deep sleep.

He never woke. Here then the invisible powei must have held him up there fast asleep, and only let go once human hands provided saftey. By this time Constable Burger was convinced that it was a native criminal whom he knew and who had a grudge against him who was responsible for this "goelery". Here we observe how in desperation the mind of a trained policeman, and a man of fair education began to regress under the strain and ignorance to the magical superstitious levels which we share with the coloureds and Africans.

He decided to go to Sophiatown to fetch a witchdoctor whom he paid five pounds. The witchdoctor confirmed his suspicions but said he needed more powerful medicines than could be obtained locally—these had to come from Zululand and more money was required to obtain this strong dope. Mr. Sadie watched how the witchdoctor sprinkled powder round the house, the window sills and thresholds. Then he took his medicine case and went to sit flat on the floor in the diningroom. He took out of his case a smallish bottle within which was a still smaller bottle. Hereafter he poured some powder into the smallest bottle with a piece of tin, and put a match to it while he was throwing the bones.

At first the bones conveyed nothing but after a while they "spoke". They said the man who was doing the mischief had powerful witchcraft medicines and the only remedy was to obtain the expensive medicine from Zululand. A week later the witchdoctor was back with the powerful medicine from Zululand. He took up his previous position flat on the floor of the diningroom.

He was as busy as before unpacking all his little bottles of medicine when the bottom of one of his bottles suddenly came away, and went spinning and whirling round and round the room, wheeling as if propelled like a wheel in flight. The witchdoctor gave a cry of terror, grabbed his case of medicines and with wild staring eyes leapt for the door and was gone. With him went the constable's money for the special medicines from Zululand.

White experts on witchcraft, and ghost catchers of all classes and races offered their help, and the curious swarmed over the place. The phenomena continued and the ghost catchers were made to look foolish. One who came with a special apparatus for catching the ghost had it pinched by the ghost and so could not use his instrument to demonstrate his powers at ghost catching. Another expert on "goelery" assured them that money was buried underneath the house, and that the person who was conducting the "goelery" wanted to have the Burger's out of the house so that he could live there and use the booty.

Constable Burger, in spite of his experience with the witchdoctor was persuaded that money was buried there, for he refused to accept the phenomena as psychic, insisting that they were caused by a physical being who utilised magical powers. The established primitive pattern of thought was more acceptable.

Then the constable broke up the floor boards and dug up the ground underneath but found no money.

After this experience Mr. Sadie informed the constable that he felt sure that Mrs. Burger was un unconscious medium and that she was ındirectly responsible for these manifestations. But the constable refused to accept this argument. He argued that his wife was the greatest sufferer from all these devilish tricks, why therefore should she allow such things to happen through her powers? He also would not agree to sending his wife away for a holiday somewhere. Then somewhat half-heartedly he agreed that Mr. Sadie could arrange for a medium to hold a seance in the house.

Mrs. Rosa Parvin of Johannesburg undertook to give a seance. She was known to have had experience with poltergeist phenomena in England. Anyway Mrs. Parvin discovered that Mrs. Burger was very mediumistic, or a sensitive psychic individual. She said certain earthbound entities were drawing on her power and creating the consternation wherever she went. During her trance her control said there were four earthbound spirits. One was a man named Hofmeyer, who years before had lived in the house. He had been married to a person named Mavis who had been divorced from her first husband and she had come with her daughter to live in Hofmeyer's home.

Hofmeyer had been a chronic alcoholic and had cruelly ill-treated the girl whenever he was under the influence of alcohol. This girl's father tried from time to time to take her away from Hofmeyer and her mother. On each occasion that he made an attempt there were terrific quarrels and fights. The girl's father eventually died in an accident and Hofmeyer drank himself to death. Mavis died in an institution for mental diseases while the daughter who had gone to a convent also died.

The drama which they had lived in their quarrels and drunken orgies continued as poltergeist phenomena. A few days later Mr. Sadie arranged another seance, and Mrs. Parvin's control said that they would try and bring Hofmeyer through the medium to assist him to gain a new insight, and release him from the bondage of his earthbound state of mind. Mr. Sadie mentioned that Mrs. Parvin was a small stoutish lady who had injured her ankle and they had to help her along as she could not put her full weight on that foot.

After the guide spoke with Mrs. Parvin while she was in a deep trance there was silence for a while. Then her hands began to open and close into clutching, claw-like movements, as if about to tear something to pieces. She got up from her chair without assistance and with her full weight on both feet, unlike she was before the trance, and advanced towards Mrs. Burger. Mr. Sadie stressed that in her normal personality Mrs. Parvin was a sensitive, tender and sweet person but on that occasion as she advanced towards Mrs. Burger her expression was one of vile depravity and wickedness. Indeed it was so terribly horrible and fiendish that they all had cold shivers at this transformation of a sweet face into something so malign.

Mr. Parvin, a shortish but powerfully built man had apparently anticipated this type of reaction, and he rose clamly and stood in the way of the advancing medium with her claw-like outstretched hands, and placed himself between her and Mrs. Burger. "Hofmeyer listen to me," he said and put out his arm to keep the medium back. "You are no longer a being with a physical body, and you cannot do harm to this lady. She's being protected by people who obtain their power from a higher source. You are powerless."

At this the medium turned to him, her small hands shot forward and grabbed him by the throat. Mr. Parvin became blue in his face and tried desperately to remove her hands. He was being strangled. Mr. Sadie said he sat there, and watched this ferocious attack. He knew he had to help, but did not know how. At once he thought that he would have to give her a knock-out blow with his fist to free her fiendish hold on her husband's throat. But how could he hit such a tender-natured kindly person as Mrs. Parvin?

But as he realized that she was overpowering her husband, he jumped up to go to his assistance, and as he rose from his deep armchair to grab her from behind, she swung round in his direction. He retreated and sank into his chair. She continued to approach with murderous groping, clutching fingers. He felt the impulse to get up and jump out of her way but found it somewhat ridiculous to run away from a little woman of her size. So he remained seated and awaited events. She came up to him and leaned forward while he continued to slide deeper into the chair as far back and away from her as possible.

He was pressing against the back of the chair and deep into the seat. There was no escape, she was now bending over him and the two deep sides of the armchair virtually hemmed him in. He could not escape except by means of some violent act. Her claw-like hands came towards his shoulders while he was trying to make himself as insignificant as possible. He was determined now to push her with all his might should she grab his throat. Then suddenly she grabbed him by the shoulders and with unbelievable strength jerked him up clean out of the chair and then threw him back into it as if he were a bundle of washing.

She repeated this feat of great strength three times, jerking him up and pushing him back into the depth of the big chair and then suddenly she let go of him, and turned round facing the sitters in a fierce challenging manner, ready for a fight with anyone. She stood for a while waiting for someone to attack her and then went back to the settee or sofa and sat down. At this stage something happened to Mrs. Burger, they thought she had fainted but soon they heard her speak incoherently. She was actually in a light trance, and according to Mrs. Parvin's spirit control the daughter who had died in the convent was trying to manifest through the mediumistic Mrs. Burger.

Evidently several seances were conducted in the home by Mrs. Parvin after which things became quiet. The earthbound spirits ceased to quarrel but Mrs. Parvin considered that it was necessary for Mrs. Burger's psychic powers to be properly developed and controlled to assist her to defend herself against these lowest astral entities. Her husband however refused to have anything to do with spiritists and Mrs. Parvin warned them that the earthbound group might return.

The house was quiet for a long time, several months in fact, and then Mrs. Burger was confronted by an apparition of a woman in her bedroom. This being wanted Mrs. Burger to accompany her and when she refused grabbed her by the arm leaving red marks which were visible the next day. After this the Burgers left the house on vacation and no more was subsequently learned about this poltergeist haunt.

Several points emerge from this most interesting account by Mr. Sadie. It is unlikely that Mrs. Burger would have initiated these physical phenomena including the hair-raising happenings to her baby. The rational explanation based on experience over ages is that Mrs. Burger was psychic as was discovered by Mrs. Parvin and suspected by Mr. Sadie. It must therefore be concluded that the purposeful and intelligent actions were performed by discarnate entities who were drawn to her because of the intensity of the field of force which she radiated.

They evidently continued to exist on the lowest degrees of the astral plane in the same mental state as they had had on earth. They were bound to the memories of the old environment in its astral reflections and hence lived the pattern of their lives unaware of the fact that they had died. The power produced by the mediumistic constitution of Mrs. Burger unbeknown to herself provided these entities with the energy system whereby they could manipulate physical objects, and abreact their own vile and aggressive impulses with occasional coarse and crude humour.

It is difficult if not well nigh impossible to advance any other explanation that will not insult one's intelligence. It is in a way amusing to study Constable Burger's prejudice against spiritism, but not against witchcraft and "goelery". The deep trance state which made it possible for Hofmeyer to use the delicate Mrs. Parvin's body with his insane strength which almost strangled her own husband showed that no conscious Mrs. Parvin had control of the situation or of her own body. The manner too in which she threw Mr. Sadie around showed that the supernormal strength was drawn not only from Mrs. Parvin but also from Mrs. Burger and possibly from others present as well.

The technique whereby an entity takes hold of another's body could to my mind only be explained on the principle of existence of the astral as the true inner personality. Once the medium enters a trance her astral body moves out of coincidence but retains its electromagnetic connections with the body cells and nerves. This connection is made possible because of the magnetic forces or neuric energy flowing along the astral silver cord. The controlling intelligence of a discarnate being hence tunes in and establishes contact with the neuric force of the silver cord and so takes possession of the body of the medium. In some such manner does it appear logical for one intelligence to replace another in the same body, apart from mere hysterical dissociations.

There is also another possibility namely that as the medium's astral body moves out of coincidence during a trance, the field of force or aura of the astral is invaded by the discarnate intelligence. This seems to me the most likely explanation. By these means it could gain control over the different energy systems and so produce speech and other manifestations. The communicating spirits or astral beings are bound to differ in ethical and aesthetic values. There will be the crude, coarse and vulgar earthbound levels of unenlightened man and those of higher spiritual values.

The system of energy employed by them however would remain basically the same. But in the case of the higher evolved consciousness the motives would produce a frequency rate of energy with the properties such as appeared in the life of my little primula. All these paranormal phenomena indicate that there is an electromagnetic characteristic about thought. It attracts and repels and seems to exercise a controlling influence over other energy systems of the human organism.

CHAPTER IV

HAUNTS

Once we accept as reasonable that there is such an inner personality as the astral, we are presented with an understanding of extrasensory faculties. The neuro-psychiatric missing link between mind and body could be found in terms of the astral.

A great deal of verbiage has been expressed on this problem of mind and body. But this approach has always excluded the role of paranormal psychic manifestations.

It is at times almost staggering to one's mind to read erudite symposiums on body and mind without a single reference to the controlled experiments and findings in psychic research.

Serious thought given to the work of the pioneers like Professor Richet's "Thirty Years of Psychic Research" for instance cannot fail to present the unprejudiced mind the reasonableness of postulating an astral personality.

The astral substance of the psyche can be considered as a system of energy which permeates all matter. But once we leave this world we enter a plane where it is the exclusive medium of existence.

In that plane it is the medium whereby the psyche expresses itself according to its mental content and emotional interests and drives at the time of death.

One could imagine a law of reflection whereby the densest layers of the astral are similar to the topography of this world. There could even be a correspondence between one's interests and mental habits in this world and the same mental habits in the lower strata of the astral.

One might even attempt to find your own social group, and the continuation of your earthly interests; even creedal in the astral world. The substance of the astral plane could be malleable to thought. That is, one might probably be able to mould the astral substance to fulfil one's needs.

The minds of Mrs. Burger's ghosts for instance were still operating with the same motivations and intentions, as though a pane of glass separated our two worlds. This symbol of a pane of glass implies that only those with astral faculties of sight like clairvoyants would be able to see through this medium between two worlds.

Those who died unconscious of a higher aspiration of life might find themselves for a time harnessed by their earthly mental habits and pleasures. These are the beings who are seen by psychic sensitives as ghosts.

They are probably not in this dimensionality at all, but in a corresponding astral reproduction of their past earthly abodes in which they are seen by the clairvoyants as if in an earthly home.

The astral vases which they smash, the astral money which they pour tinkling down the stairs are never found as physical objects, because they happen in the astral dimensionality. The psychic sensitive sees with astral sight and hears with astral hearing and could provide the power for low-grade astral intelligences to become poltergeists.

So we can attribute all our extrasensory perceptions including precognition and even telekinesis so common to poltergeists to the powers—supraphysical of the astral body.

Let science establish the truth of the astral body, and its energy systems and biology, medicine, psychiatry and neurology will be enabled to reveal some profound mysteries of life.

It could be that the astral plane or dimensionality meaning hereby a state of existence, is also revolving relative to the earth plane so that occasions occur when there is coincidence between the astral topography and the terrestrial topography.

The question arises whether periodic ghostly manifestations or haunts do not occur during such coincidences of the two dimensionalities. These could be moments of strong overflow from the astral because of old earthly interests and memories.

The astral itself could be a substance which not only transcends the physical, but also has the capacity for registering impressions and retaining memories in the nature of vibrations or thought patterns.

The faculty of psychometry or psychoscopy seems to me to be much better explained as a form of astral perception, than just as vibrations from an object.

Psychometry does not appear to be dependent on information from discarnate spirits, but seems to be a faculty of the human mind, albeit not overtly active in most people.

The phenomena perceived by holding an object in the hand are not lifeless. They usually unfold a rich colourful process of someone's past experience with all the emotional components whether tragedy, sorrow or joy.

If therefore astral energy retaining associations of the memories of a person were contained in a brooch, coin, or pocket book belonging to someone, those astral memories with all their rich associations will again be available to the astral perceptive faculties of the psychic individual.

Many a life story can be told from an object. The witchdoctor Solomon Daba used to give me some fascinating descriptions of people by merely handling objects belonging to them.

The astral world and its psychic powers have its common frontier with the physical, in fact the physical could be but a peel of which it is the fruit.

When man is so superstitiously inclined as to abhor these deeper facets of life, whose tenants we are, and so readily associate evil influences with the next world, because of contact in ignorance with the densest beings of astral life, it is refreshing to relate the story of the appearance of the Jewish Rabbi to a little boy.

This account is authentically given by Mr. Sadie. The incident was communicated to him by a colleague and a friend of his, Mr. R. Hendriks a well-known Afrikaans detective story writer.

The Hendriks family moved into a flat in Johannesburg from their previous home in Northcliffe. One evening his wife had to go somewhere urgently to keep an appointment, but they had no one to leave in the flat with their little son of six years. They did not at all like the idea of leaving him alone, but had no alternative except to wait until he was asleep and then to go by car as quickly as possible. They felt that this would be the best solution because he was a heavy sleeper, and hardly ever woke during the night. He fell asleep and they slipped out quietly to keep the appointment. On their return half-an-hour later they found the little fellow sitting up in bed wide awake.

"Where were you"? he asked. "I woke and called and called to you, but there was no answer." And what did you do then?" asked his parents. "At first I cried," he said, "but then an uncle (oom) came out behind the curtain there and said to me "Don't cry big man, your Pappa and Mamma will be here any minute."

"What sort of an uncle," (oom) asked his completely astounded father. "What did he look like?" "Oh," said the little fellow: "He wore spectacles and had on a long black frock (robe) and on his head was a small black hat." "And then?" went on the father, "what did you do?" "Oh we played. The uncle was very funny and made me laugh."

"But where is he now?" asked his father. "He disappeared behind the curtain there and said you would be arriving." Mrs. Hendriks laughed and believed that her little boy had imagined and fabricated the whole story, and added that "he had his father's talent." They dismissed the whole episode until some days later someone who knew the flat casually remarked about an old Jewish Rabbi who had lived and died in that flat.

This pricked Mr. Hendriks' curiosity and the next morning he asked the African who had cleaned these flats for a long time whether he knew about the Rabbi, and the servant confirmed that he had died there and had worn spectacles, a long black robe and a small black cap.

Here then the Rabbi from behind the pane of astral glass stepped into the astral vision of the little boy and with paternal kindness amused him until his parents returned.

Another interesting statement from Mr. Sadie concerned a clairvoyant gentleman who was awakened from sleep by someone who came to tell him about a great shock sustained by his brother's daughter of twelve that evening.

She evidently walked out of the house to do some task for her mother, when in front of the kitchen door something barged against her and flung her aside for quite a few yards, and on the spot of this impact the members of the family saw a ball of light move backwards and forwards for a while.

The clairvoyant gentleman whose name Mr. Sadie withheld for certain reasons, immediately left for his brother's farm. He found this girl of twelve in bed, mute with shock and fear, and unable to move her one arm and leg. He could not get a word out of her. She seemed in a stupor.

He decided to investigate accompanied by the girl's father, and at once he saw the cause of the girl's fright. An old man with dark glasses and a bent back with a stick in his hand went past the kitchen door.

He followed the phantom to a little stream a long way from the homestead near an avenue of fig trees. Here the phantom turned and went back the way he had come, using his stick as he walked. He passed in front of the kitchen door and about two hundred yards farther on disappeared near the ruins of an old building.

When this description was given to the people of the house they immediately recognised him as an old blind man who during his earth life regularly everyday walked from the house to the little stream and back past the kitchen towards the ruins.

The psychic gentleman with his clairvoyant faculty decided to obtain telepathic communication with the old man's astral being. He conveyed to him the necessity of changing his habits. He must have succeeded because from that time the phantom was never seen again.

This account clearly illustrates how a habit of mind continued to operate in the astral environment; a reproduction of his previous surroundings. For years he had walked there behind his pane of glass separating him from the world of physical life, and then one evening as he passed the kitchen this young girl—prepubertal and in all probability psychic and therefore surrounded by a powerful field of force or aura, acted as a magnet and drew the old man's astral form into contact with her own.

His mind was repeating an earthly habit. When he collided with the girl there occurred something very similar to a flash of lightning, even including the fireball of electromagnetic discharge, leaving the girl in a state of psychic shock and exhaustion for a while.

Someone sent me a copy of the *Suid Afrikaanse Stem*, wherein a Mr. Piet de Klerk described a story of haunting associated with a doll. A certain Mrs. Barnes of Barberton had a little daughter Johanna eight years old who had had polio, and during her stay in hospital her other sister Hester, seventeen years of age, had been killed in an accident.

When Johanna came home her mother took her to see her sister Hester's grave, and while there Johanna said Hester was very lonely lying there alone in the grave. She wanted her mother to leave her beautiful big doll on Hester's grave to keep her company. When her mother said that her doll would be stolen if left on the grave, Johanna suggested that they bury the doll there to keep Hester company. It is quite plain that to Johanna her dolly was possessed of life and interest.

Her little mind gave the doll all these qualities and so she believed it would equally be a companion to her sister whom she thought was lying alive in the grave. This shows that children do not understand the lifelessness of death. Their own animation is always projected on to the objects of their thoughts especially where it concerns someone known in life.

Mrs. Barnes did not decide on Johanna's suggestion to bury the doll and before long Johanna died of pneumonia. Mrs. Barnes had to leave for Pretoria and so offered Johanna's almost life-sized doll to Mr. and Mrs. Trent for safe keeping.

They placed the doll on a chair in the sittingroom. One evening Mrs. Trent went to the kitchen for a drink of water and in the dusk as she passed through the sittingroom her eye fell on the doll. To her amazement she saw a sort of misty figure of a little girl sitting on the arm of the easy-chair stroking the hair of the doll with her right hand. While Mrs. Trent was staring at this vision the little girl looked up at her and smiled sweetly. Realizing this to be a supernormal phenomenon Mrs. Trent gave one scream of terror and fled to her husband. He pooh-poohed the idea as nonsense and went to find nothing more than the huge doll staring at him with its wide-open blue eyes.

About three evenings later he walked to the kitchen and saw the doll sitting on the settee. On his return from the kitchen he looked again, and there sat the little girl as his wife had seen her, gently stroking the doll's hair and smiling sweetly at him. He felt his hair rise on end and he went to his wife to tell her about his experience. They decided to get rid of the doll at the first opportunity and so hid it behind a wardrobe. When Mrs. Barnes returned the doll was immediately handed back to her. The Trents did not want it anywhere near them.

Mrs. Barnes placed the doll under a sheet on the bed, because a small baby who had looked at it had started crying almost hysterically as if terrified. Another twelve-year old daughter of Mrs. Barnes named Bokkie saw the sheet moving over the doll as if the doll were deeply asleep and breathing. She pulled off the sheet and saw the doll staring at her with her huge blue eyes. Bokkie screamed and ran away in terror. The doll looked alive. Her little girl Bokkie, according to Mrs. Barnes, was deathly pale and terrified.

Then some time later Mrs. Barnes was reading by a dim light, and at once she felt an impulse to look at the doll. While she sat watching it lying on its back on the bed it made several attempts to sit up, but fell back each time. Mrs. Barnes closed her eyes and opened them wide to make sure that she was actually seeing the doll trying to sit up, and there was the doll doing just what she first saw and staring at her with huge, blue glowing eyes as if she wanted to say something.

Mrs Barnes became terrified, her hair stood on end and she ran screaming from the room. She ended the interview with Mr. de Klerk by saying, "If only I knew what is happening. Why does the doll haunt us? Is it my Johanna who has returned from the dead to play with her doll? What must I do? What must I do?" The story closed on this anguished cry of the mother whose mind had been confused by the lack of enlightenment in spiritual upbringing, and the sinister meaning which superstition and ignorance had woven into these tragedies of the human mentality.

The picture is one of a dominating affection of the little girl for her dolly. This attraction was so powerful that her astral self was drawn to it and to her home. In the presence of people she absorbed sufficient of their radiations to become so dense that she could be seen and even smile, showing her pleasure at being able to play with her doll.

No doubt the radiations of her twelve-year old sister Bokkie added to the power so that Johanna could actually make the doll breathe and move the sheet. That is if Bokkie had not imagined the movement. But Mrs. Barnes also must have provided power for Johanna to try and make her dolly sit up.

One could imagine this little girl on the other side of my pane of astral glass trying to convey to people by means of her doll that she was very much alive and enjoying her games with her dolly which had given her so much pleasure during life. Yet all we found was the anguished note of the mother's interview, showing the dark regions of our scientific atomic age.

The following account of a haunt was sent to me by Mr. E. Silk of Johannesburg, who was an Anglican Minister resident on the alluvial diamond diggings at Windsorton during 1915. This place is about forty miles from Kimberley.

I quote from his letter.

"I used to conduct services there once a fortnight, and as one of the services was a late evening one, I had to stay at Klipdam over Sunday night, returning to Windsorton on Monday morning, by bicycle.

"The small population consisted of a number of diggers, a diamond buyer or two, the magistrate and the police. The whole country round about was desolate and there was hardly anything to be seen except heaps of stones and rocks. Klipdam was a desolate place. I usually had supper on Sunday with a parishioner and went to sleep at the hotel, which was a wood-and-iron building.

"On several occasions, as soon as I got into bed, I used to hear a sound outside the room, as of a very strong wind getting up. I remember on two occasions that I got up and looked out of the window to see if I could see any movement in the trees, but no movement was visible so I went back to bed.

"Then the room used to begin to sound as though it was shaking though I personally felt no movement. The shaking sounded as if the roof and iron walls were shaking violently. I cannot remember being at all afraid about it.

"Then after a time of this noise of wind and shaking, I used to feel what appeared to be a large flabby hand making its way round the back of my neck until it reached my throat. When this took place I felt as though something was trying to possess me. If my eyes were open I could not shut them. If shut, I could not open them, nor open my mouth to speak.

"While I was thus held the shaking continued and became more and more violent, and I was kept in this state for about ten minutes. Then gradually the flabby hand would withdraw the way it came, via the back of my neck, the noise of the shaking would gradually subside and then I was able to move again. As a finale to all this, just as I felt released from whatever it was that was holding me, I used to hear a very loud crash in the room, as though everything moveable in the room had crashed in a heap in the middle of the room. As soon as I could move I used to jump up, light the candle, and on looking round found everything in order. There was never anything that could have accounted for the crash.

"I do not know whether the hotel is still standing. Klipdam itself has I understand come to an end. I mentioned these experiences to the proprietor at the time. He asked me not to say anything or repeat them to others, and informed me that other people who had stayed at the hotel had related similar experiences.

"This was not the end; I asked one of the parishioners to give me sleeping accommodation at her house. There was only a stretcher available on which I slept outside under the stars. I was getting tired of having my sleep disturbed at the hotel and so sought other accommodation. The same experience however followed me and I cannot just remember how it happened when I slept on the stretcher. Certainly the hand came round the back of my neck as usual, and I was unable to move for some little time. What I cannot remember here is whether there was any sound of wind or noise of shaking.

"This person then went away on holiday and I asked the magistrate whether he could put me up. He said his wife was on holiday and he had a spare room. I went there and hoped to be secure from the 'thing'. I lay awake but hearing noises I was somewhat fearful as my room was at the farthest end of a large old rambling house. However on getting up to investigate I discovered that a white horse was shuffling along the verandah and came past the window.

"I returned to bed and tried to sleep, but at about midnight to my horror the experience began again as at the hotel—the wind, the shaking and the hand and subsequent inability to move. It lasted about the usual time but the crash seemed bigger than usual. I immediately jumped out of bed, lit the candle but found everything in order.

"I felt on this occasion that things were getting a bit too disturbing and at 4 a.m. I dressed and as it was still dark I went to the police station and found that a mounted policeman was leaving at that time for Windsorton. I accompanied him on my bicycle. I did not return to Klipdam after that and left for England. I never saw anything during these experiences but certainly felt the flabby hand.

"When I returned from England I went to reside at Batlharos, a mission station near Kuruman, living there for seven-and-a-half years. One night I heard the noise of the wind as I had heard it at Klipdam. My first thought was that I was going to have another experience, but the wind passed overhead. The facts as I have stated are perfectly true."

Here then we have an account of a reputable and reliable witness. I have given the Reverend Silk's experience in full detail, because of its most interesting features, which make it possible to venture an explanation as comprehensible as words will allow.

His experience illustrates what happens when a drama is enacted by an earthbound being in the astral world, or on the other side of the pane of glass of that dimensionality. The noise of the strong wind getting up was not in this world, but in the astral because the trees outside showed no movement. Then the shaking as though the wood-and-iron walls were shaking violently and yet nothing moved physically. So all the violence and shaking were taking place in another dimensionality and not in this physical world.

But the Reverend Silk's consciousness was turned into the astral world and unbeknown to himself he had psychic qualities, and the power to radiate an aura of such intensity that his astral energies became conjoined with those of the astral world proper, making it possible for some paranoidal depraved earthbound entity in the densest regions of the astral to re-enact some murderous drama which had taken place on a stormy night at Klipdam.

Was it someone in a drunken state who tried to rob someone else of his diamonds? In any case he was not powerful. The hands were soft and flabby. Nevertheless the original earthly event which became transplanted on to the astral, activated the consciousness, so that the motive and impulse continued to live in bondage to its depraved thought-world. Hence whenever someone with a strong aura or field of force came within that locality the astral spirit was drawn to that person to reincarnate his original impulses.

What is of interest is the cataleptic state in which the Reverend Silk found himself. This is strongly suggestive of an attempt to go into a trance, for he even felt that the being wanted to possess him. It supports my contention that the Reverend Silk was mediumistic.

This phenomena of a depraved astral assault also happened to others, and the proprietor evidently wanted it kept a secret for business reasons. Perhaps he knew the story behind this astral drama. In any case it is my opinion that only those who could manifest an aura of sufficient power to establish contact with the astral world could have been the victims of the entity with the flabby hands. It was actually the Reverend Silk's astral throat which he was trying to strangle.

Another communication received from Mrs. E. C. Blaxland of London is of special interest to those who know St. Mary's Collegiate Church in Port Elizabeth. Her husband was rector of St. Mary's from 1935.

Mrs. Blaxland who is psychic was at that time both clairvoyant and clairaudient. Not only could she perceive astral beings with her astral sight, but she could hear with her astral faculty of hearing.

It is of significance to note that sometimes one astral faculty is prominent in a physical personality, while the other astral channels of perception are dormant. The Reverend Silk for instance had astral hearing or clairaudience well developed, and even of touch, but as far as his astral sight was concerned he had no developed capacity for clairvoyant vision.

In the case of Mrs. Barnes and the Trent family with the blue-eyed doll, we find that some degree of astral sight was present in all of them. These anomalies indicate that astral perceptivity not only varies as extrasensory perception, but that there is more of it in one or other faculty of certain persons and frequently dormant capacities in others.

Mrs. Blaxland kindly wrote to me as follows :

"We arrived at Port Elizabeth on August 1st, 1935 and were met by a party of about a dozen people who came on board to welcome us. We told them that our furniture would arrive a few days later, and that we would go to an hotel until the rectory was ready with all our belongings in it. There seemed to be some hesitation before some of the party told us that the rectory was not fit for us to live in for two reasons. First reason was that it was excessively damp, and the second was that it was haunted.

We told them that we were quite prepared to make the best of it but they were adamant. They told us that during the interregum one of the assistant clergy had been sleeping there to try it out before putting the new rector in it to live. He had been very disturbed at night due to inexplicable noises and he had had his bedclothes pulled off. The result of this was that we settled in a flat until a new rectory should be built. No one seemed to be willing or able to give any explanation of all the happenings. We could not help wondering how it was that the previous rector had been able to live in such a house for many years.

St. Mary's Collegiate Church was a fine one, and it had a magnificent organ. It also had a first-class organist and choir. As I had played the organ for many years I was allowed to practise on this lovely instrument, and to play for services when Mr. G. the organist was away on his annual holiday.

The organ was a five manual one, it was a great joy to play on it as it had such a beautiful tone. I noticed that whenever I played there was always someone in the Church listening to the music. He moved about in the choir and sometimes sat in one of the stalls. Several times he came into the organ loft and stood behind me, silently slipping out while I was still playing.

I mentioned this to my husband as I like to be alone when I am practising. He said that it was best to leave well alone and if the visitor enjoyed the music it did no harm to have him there. I did not mention this to anyone else as many people used the Church for private prayers. I admit that the presence of someone standing close to me when I played was a little eerie as I never managed to catch sight of his face.

One day my husband came in after an afternoon's visiting and told me that he had visited an old lady who would not come to Church because she was afraid of meeting the ghost. She insisted that other people had seen it and that she was not going to run risks.

My husband inquired of the verger if there was any truth in the story that the Church was haunted. He at once said that he was surprised; he had heard nothing about it before we arrived. He said that he often saw the "old man" and that he came into the Lady Chapel almost every day. Sometimes he would kneel at the high altar and at other times he would wander about in the choir or go into the organ loft. We thought no more of this as nothing ever happened to cause undue trouble and in any case we could do nothing about it.

One Sunday evening a couple asked us to drive them down to Church. They said that it was their wedding anniversary and that they would like to come. (They were very delightful parishioners who did not come regularly to Church). When we got into the Church they sat with me, about a third of the way down the nave from the front. It was an immense Church and there were very large congregations. After the service they sat with me in the car waiting for my husband.

While we were waiting our friend whom I will call Mr. X suddenly said :— "What's this new bit of ritual you have here?" I did not know what he could be referring to, but he continued :— "Well, why does one of the clergy stand in front of the altar during the anthem?" I told him that I was following the score of the anthem and had not looked up at all, but in any case my husband was the only person there as the rest of the staff were at outstations.

But Mr. X insisted that he had seen the man come in through the door beyond the choir stalls on the north side. From there he walked to the middle of the choir facing the altar. There he had stayed all through the anthem and had gone out of the door by which he had come in.

I asked him to describe this priest and as he did so I began to realize whom he might have seen, so I asked him if he would recognize him if he saw his photograph? We asked them home and I made sure from my husband that no other clergy had been there.

I proceeded to get a history of Port Elizabeth which had been given to us, and I showed him the photograph of the late rector who had been at St. Mary's during the whole of his ministry, and as a young man before he had been ordained, a period of seventy years or more.

At once Mr. X said that he was the person who had come into the Church during the anthem. After this we made many inquiries, and we came across others who had seen him. Among them was one who told us that the late rector had been devoted to music and had given the organ to the Church.

He also said that the late rector had used the door beyond the choir stalls a great deal. During our time in Port Elizabeth it was never used at all. The place where he had been standing before the altar was his grave. Sometime after we had left we heard that the Bishop of the Diocese had been asked to exorcise the Church and that he had done so.

We were sorry to hear this, as a good spirit who loves a place and who is drawn to come back to it can do no harm to anyone, and indeed would wish them well; if he is cast out of it where does he go? There was a peaceful atmosphere at St. Mary's which he so often visited and if I ever come back I should miss him."

I can endorse Mrs. Blaxland's impression of the peace and calm atmosphere which reigns in St. Mary's Church. I have often walked in there during the day to disengage my mind from the turmoil and problems of the world outside.

But apart from the pleasure and peace which the discarnate rector found in St. Mary's his astral visits do raise certain interesting aspects of spirit behaviour. His was not an automatic performance of a shell of his being, or a mere photograph or thought-form of habitual memories and actions, those mental robots in which certain people find solace and an easy plausible explanation for ghosts and haunts. No, to all intents and purposes he appeared at selected times and showed curiosity as well as pleasure at having a new organist.

He occupied various positions in the Church during Mrs. Blaxland's playing and even came to stand behind her as if looking at the music. These were intelligent and purposive actions, and when there was a large congregation he came in and stood facing the altar over his grave while the anthem was being sung.

His sense of proprietorship was also in evidence when one of the assistant clergy slept in the old rectory. He came and pulled the bedclothes off his colleague. He was apparently annoyed at a stranger taking the liberties of sleeping in his house without his permission or knowledge. He was indeed wedded to his Church and his rectory and somehow resented any intrusion of his home.

This then appears to have been his attitude of mind, which in turn reflects that his spiritual consciousness was somewhat stultified. He was indeed most devoted from a churchianic point of view. But could one say that this was a religion which stimulated aspiration for spiritual evolution, and for progress into those mystic regions of life which our earthly minds are unable to conceive? His religious aspirations apparently did not embrace a higher development of consciousness, by means of which mind would shed the petals of earthly values, so that its inner revelations may become realizations.

If these qualities were the dynamic forces of his religious feelings, his reverence and especially his sense of wonder, then his entrance into the astral after death would have actuated him to reach for planes other than habitual earthly values and habits.

If the exorcism by the Bishop made the discarnate rector realize his sojourn on the lower strata of the astral, and awakened his consciousness to the need for seeking his spiritual pleasures at higher levels, then the Bishop indeed rendered him a service. Exorcism after all is exclusively prayer and therefore a form of telepathic communication with the discarnate being, which is intended to bring him to a new realization of his state of mind and his habits and desires.

One is reminded of the case of the blind old man who barged into the young girl, as mentioned by Mr. Sadie. In that case the clairvoyant gentleman communicated with him telepathically and the astral being of the old man woke, as it were, from his dream of earthly habits and probably immediately adjusted himself to the true conditions and enjoyments of his astral potentialities and faculties.

The mind of man can therefore become anchored to this world, as if magnetised by his interests and habits and hence however pious not reach those subtle degrees of abstract thought and feeling which characterise a spiritual consciousness and its endeavours.

Mrs. Blaxland's account of the ghost of St. Mary's reveals therefore that even a clergyman could be earth-bound and suggests that orthodox religion should carefully re-examine its conceptions and methods of instruction.

I have in my possession a large number of letters in Afrikaans on psychic experiences. All of them carry the stamp of deep sincerity and honesty and many of them reveal the inner search of minds which are unable to find in their religious practices and beliefs an explanation of these experiences.

In fact, they give the impression that these matters are tabooed by the church. A brief translation of the following letter tells its own story :— "I am an elder in the church and a deeply religious man who through experience with supernormal phenomena have convinced myself that the soul of man survives death.

I have often seen those who have died during the day as well as during the night, and although the teachings of my church interpret these things otherwise I will follow my own conscience and inner directives.

As a boy of fourteen years I one day accompanied a man on his horse-and-cart to a farm where he had business. Having outspanned the horses at our destination, I remained sitting next to the cart because I did not want to intrude on the company of adults.

While sitting there I noticed a huge earthen-dam wall near the south side of the house. I just sat thinking of nothing in particular when I noticed a lovely little girl some twenty yards from the dam wall. She stood and looked at me and I looked at her. She had on a white Boer "kappie" (bonnet), a blue dress, white socks and black shoes. Suddenly she turned and walked towards the dam wall, where there were a few large stones and at that spot she disappeared over the dam wall.

I noticed that the child was floating in the air rather than walking, but I attributed this to the heat of the day. I did not then think of a spirit, but of a child in the flesh. My curiosity aroused I went to look what had become of the little girl. I found the dam bone-dry and no child anywhere. I looked all over but could not find her.

When I returned to the cart I found that another cart had outspanned in my absence and a boy of my own age was sitting there. We started to talk and I said to him that I felt uncomfortable there because it seemed to me that the people of the farm had no children. Then he told me that they had had one little girl, but she had been drowned in that very dam, having fallen in one day just where the big stones were.

In 1932 at the age of sixteen years I was working for a man who trained race horses and he had three jockeys, two coloured and a native. It was 4 p.m. and I came out of the house and saw a horse and rider galloping up to a farm gate. At the gate the rider dismounted; he was a native man; he opened the gate, led the horse through, shut the gate and mounted and was off at a gallop down the hill. I thought it was one of our boys and went down to the dam to meet the rider and the horse, and as I neared the gate I could see the rider's head, it was just visible above the high land bobbing up and down, up and down.

But all at once I saw the rider and horse disappear near a tree. I thought they had had a fall and I ran to the spot where there were thorn bushes, but found nothing. I spoke about this strange experience and an old native man told me that during the Anglo-Boer war a native was a spy for the British, and he came along there on horseback one afternoon but the Boers were waiting for him and shot both him and the horse. The old native and others dug a huge hole and buried both rider and horse near the tree and the thorn bushes. Then they showed me the grave; it was marked with stones.

From that time I have had many experiences and am aware of telepathic communications from those who have passed on when there was a need to communicate ideas."

In the following case the phantom was seen by the writer and his companion. He said that it was just after the Anglo-Boer war and they were very poor. The sheep from two farms were herded together in the Clanwilliam district.

There were four young lads who looked after the sheep and at midday they used to herd the sheep and drive them to a water-hole for drinking. One day he and his companion were on one side of the flock, while the other two lads were some distance away on the other side of the sheep.

They were about one hundred yards apart. Suddenly he and his companion saw a tall man clothed in white, almost like a long nightgown, walking along with the other two fellows, alongside the flock and then as they approached the others the tall white person disappeared.

They were naturally puzzled and questioned the other two as to whether they too had seen this man but they had no idea that they had been accompanied by anyone. They searched the spot where the figure had disappeared and to their astonishment noticed for the first time a raised grave with stones on it. When they told the story to their parents they learned that during the Anglo-Boer war the British shot a coloured man at that spot and they buried him there.

Another lady described a peculiar dream—she never had any psychic experiences except this vivid dream. She wrote :—"Shortly after moving into our present home, which we rent, I started dreaming of a little black dog—what breed I could not determine, except that it was a small type. This dog would run in at the front door, through to the bedroom and stand up on its hind legs against my bed panting; then would look around all over and just walk away again. The dream was so clear and graphic that I would wake up in a bath of perspiration. On waking I could, time and again, actually hear the pitter-patter of his little paws as he walked away.

The frequency of this dream worried me so much that I mentioned it to the owner of the house. To my surprise she told me that while living in the house she had owned a little black Scots terrier for fourteen years. He was buried on the premises. From the moment that I thought of this doggie in this way the troublesome dream ceased and has not occurred since."

It is my belief that these phantoms were all seen by means of astral sight, and they appeared as if the scenes were being enacted on a parallel plane. What is the purpose of this repetition of an event? Does it not appear as if the impulses, the dynamics and the propulsions of life which preceded death, were still wrapped up in the same habit of consciousness as a memory which enslaved the individual?

It seems almost that after one has crossed into the unseen world, thought continues to play off the energy which life's transition had brought over from the previous existence. Is there a psychological factor, which loosens this thought from its moorings, when perceived by the astral sight and the understanding of one on this side of the grave? Are these haunts, phantoms and visions forms of astral abreaction brought about by the life impulse itself to promote progression by means of developing inner awareness? Maybe there is a psychopathology of death quite unknown to us, and submerged beneath the layers of our primitive mentalities, and their magical beliefs. Perhaps we must not exclude undue scepticism.

The little Scots terrier was perhaps looking for his mistress on the astral plane. He used to run through the house—stand on his short hind legs with his panting red tongue and beady eyes, looking for her familiar touch and affection. And then when those bonds of love were not gratified he wandered away pit-a-pat, pit-a-pat, back into the doggie regions of the astral.

Mrs. van der Heever who dreamed this dream so strikingly, and repeatedly, did not know that when her astral self was out of coincidence with her physical body, she was astrally in the world in which the astral Scots terrier was repeating his joyous return to his mistress. There is an element of sadness in his little pitter-patter that died away without the love which he came to seek.

A Mrs. S. G. van Aarde of Pretoria wrote to tell me about her extraordinary experiences. She used to perceive events that have happened or were about to happen while not in full consciousness, but in a state of sleepiness—as though she was just about to drop off to sleep. At that moment she could penetrate into another world, and see writing as on a sheet of paper which moved to and fro before her sight. It was as though she was looking at writing just beneath an inch of water. She could see persons dressed to the minutest detail and every word spoken was registered and remembered. Before she moved to another house, long before they even knew about a suitable home, she would see it in detail, including the colours and other features of the building.

Then her husband and her mother died, and she moved back to her old home. From that time the most extraordinary happenings took place. There were noises, movement of objects, rappings under the table and footsteps all over the place. On the occasions when she visited her next-door neighbour in the evening, they would tell her that her bedroom was brightly lit, and when she went back to investigate the light would go out. She left this house and nothing happened in the other homes where she lived, but after a while she longed to return because of memories and at once the whole process started again.

She decided to endure the phenomena thinking that perhaps the spirits of her husband and her mother were using these means to prove their survival and to her amazement from the moment that she thought of them as existing and capable of receiving her thoughts all manifestations ceased and she lived quietly and happily in her old house.

Some people might say that the energy became exhausted in the course of time and this could be the reason for the cessation of the haunting, or one could imagine that the aura of Mrs. van Aarde became less potent as a medium to be affected by these impulses from beyond. Whatever reason one accepts, the fact remains that her changed attitude of mind played an important role. These dramatic changes in haunts do suggest that there is a particular psychology behind the haunt, like a mental force requiring expression and what I have called abreaction could be the chief motive for haunting manifestations.

The term abreaction is employed by medical psychologists for the process of releasing a repressed emotion by reliving in imagination the original experience. Now if we accept the inner personality as formed of an astral waveband of energy, we can expect that this being is destined to new adaptations after death in a new dimensionality of life. Once we agree to this conception we can imagine that earthly thought patterns and emotions which cannot find full expression and gratify their needs over there, and which still remain as stresses or charges in the mind, will have to be relived somehow.

Hence these impulses could initiate a series of activities in which the past is relived, and so indirectly serve as a sort of psychic catharsis, whereby as I have mentioned before these impulses inappropriate for the new dimensionality could be worked off and dissipated, as it were.

Not only was Mrs. van Aarde psychic but her two sons have a

peculiar olfactory psychic sense, that is, they experienced a peculiar smell as a premonition of death. Her husband had dream previsions and described to her that he dreamed his dead body was placed in an ambulance. While they did this a number of children crowded round, and the policeman present chased the children away for being indecently curious. Her husband was a soldier and well at the time, but the next day he died suddenly, and his body was placed in an ambulance with children crowding round; then a policeman came along and chased them away.

Mrs. M. A. Berry of Joubert Park, Johannesburg described a phantom of a woman in grey, but she could not see the head, nor the arms and legs. It was a grey apparition floating along as if draped in a long frock and with hooded head, so that no face was discernible. In fact, it was a featureless being, rather more a grey cloudy column resembling a person draped from head to foot in some soft material like tulle. Mrs. Berry first saw this apparition in 1950 and since then has noticed that the advent of the apparition was always associated with bad news or death concerning the family. "I just get creepy and goosey when it appears.

"Once I went to look at ahouse to rent and as I entered it I felt this sinister presence. I took my uncle there for his opinion, and we were no sooner in the house when he said 'Let us get out,' which we did as hastily as we could and locked the door behind us. Even to this day I feel and see the apparition before I hear of bad news, and when it appears I am distressed for I know something unpleasant is about to happen."

I have had numerous letters from people about phantoms of some sort or other appearing as visions in diverse forms and shapes. There were people who had foreseen their own deaths, and others who had been warned by an apparition which strangely seemed to act as an announcer. There were people who had seen a vision of a deceased friend smiling pleasantly weeks or days before their own deaths. The latter could be interpreted as continued friendship bonds, with precognition on the part of the astral friend, that the earthly one was coming over, and so because of aura power available at that moment, the astral friend briefly manifested, as much as to say "I shall meet you."

Although the sensory consciousness might not realize the true significance, the astral consciousness within and subconscious would be sure to know what it all means, and hence would recall the memory and so obtain reassurance of the transition when the deceased person entered the astral consciousness after death. But the case of Mrs. Berry and many many others of a similar nature almost reminds one of the Greek concept of Thanatos as the personification of death.

Is this part of a universal law of self-preservation in which the inner consciousness of man is constantly on the alert for the moment of eternal transition, which we call death? In those in whom these extrasensory faculties of the astral are less hampered by the physical energies, than is usual or normal, these astral perceptivities could become aware of intended phenomena. These could be brought about by discarnate beings who for some reason or other feel themselves impelled to appear to a psychic sensitive such as Mrs. Berry serving as a warning symbol or apparition.

The reason might lie in some morbid preoccupation of the discarnate being during earth life, or perhaps could imply that the deceased suffered misfortune or disaster on earth by ignoring her own premonitions or intuitions. Her astral mind could be obsessed with this idea and so attempt to rectify its mistakes by warning others to whom she could be drawn.

I am strongly inclined to think that there are simple psychological reasons for these happenings, and that they are often quite similar to known psychological mechanisms or motivated by thoughts of an obsessive nature as known in psychiatry. It is a sort of self-inflicted condition or pattern of thought which breaks through on the astral into a form of morbid self-expression.

Many of the stories about haunts showed a periodicity which does suggest that the energy systems must be favourable for the manifestation, and as I have mentioned, periodicity could mean coincidence of lowest astral topography with that of the earth. But this condition would require that there is someone in that locality at that time to furnish the necessary radiative power for the required density to cause the phenomena.

The behaviour of animals, especially dogs and horses in the presence of such concentrated supernormal atmospheres indicate that the astral manifestation is a reality, which they perceive as unusual and having disturbing vibrations. The same effects that we feel as gooseflesh and hair standing on end.

Mr. C. D. de Winnaar wrote to me from the Orange Free State about a haunt in his house, but he wanted advice and was very worried. He moved to a house outside the town because of his two huge watchdogs which were so ferocious and fearless that he had a great deal of trouble in the town with his neighbours. In view of this trouble he decided he would rather move away to another house than part with his two dogs. He said that no stranger would venture near his home. They were always on guard going round and round his property, especially at night.

They were no sooner in the new house than the dogs barked and chased round the house the whole night long. He got up several times but could not see a thing. Later he kept them in an enclosed stoep but they howled and fought to get into the house. They were even trying to scratch their way though the door to get into the house.

One night while the dogs were in uproar his wife stood up and looked through the window, and saw a ball of light floating along and then disappearing into the ground. "I was asleep at that moment and actually dreamed of seeing a ball of light coming from a church tower clock to the ground. I woke up and saw my wife at the window, and she told me what she had seen and this was similar to my dream.

We have a little daughter of eleven who has to walk through the veld for some distance to school. A few mornings after we had seen the lights, she left as usual for school with her school bag. She was hardly gone when my wife heard the child screaming in distress, and as she ran outside she found her in a state of collapse and deathly pale running wildly towards the house.

When she calmed down but could hardly speak, she kept pointing at a certain tree some distance from the house. After some time she described how she was walking along absent-mindedly and suddenly saw an apparition in front of her. He turned his head towards her and she saw that he had a very red face with two deep dark eyes. He had a head and shoulders but not the lower half of his body.

The dogs were still kept on the stoep, but behaved in a most terrified manner every night. Now a few nights ago my eldest daughter of eighteen years walked some distance with a friend who was leaving, and she turned at the gate about two hundred yards from the house. She was walking along humming a tune and not thinking of anything in particular. She came to the same tree where her little sister had seen the half-man with his red face and big dark eyes. Then as she came near the tree, she suddenly became aware of a semi-transparent cloud-like figure of a person who produced a hand which he put out very slowly in her direction, as if he wanted to shake hands. She received a terrific fright and started screaming in an uncontrolled manner whilst running for home as fast as she could, completely beside herself. She almost had convulsions from fright as her body shook, shivered and trembled.

Since then we have seen the light several times and I have seen the grey transparent apparition in front of my door. We have also heard an agonising cry inside the house in the presence of strangers as if a voice was crying deep within a cave. On one occasion, the cry changed to speech, but not one of us could make out what was said. The voice lasted about three minutes, and then stopped at once, but during this time my two ferocious dogs stormed through the kitchen door and hid cowering under my bed from where I had to drag them out. Can you please give me advice?"

Everyone will agree that there is no simple advice, but one can be sure that several members of that family were psychic, and were capable of radiating an impressionable field of force. The phenomena suggests that somewhere on the astral plane there is an individual who could have been shot near or hanged from that tree. Some catharsis or abreaction of that drama was taking place on the astral as reflected and registered memories of the world. All these haunts and happenings obey laws which are beyond our present most advanced scientific knowledge, but the haunt on Mr. de Winnaar's place was fundamentally gruesome and terrifying even to the dogs. It had the characteristics of a re-enactment of a tragedy—what I call a process of astral catharsis seen only by those on earth capable of astral vision.

The dogs therefore had good astral sight or extrasensory perception. I suppose the remedy for these manifestations in the first place is to recognise that there is a dynamic factor at the back of them. Secondly that there is an intelligent factor as well, and that a purposive trend, an intention in fact cannot be excluded. There was variation in method of presentation and manifestation, and one cannot help but sense that there was an unconscious appeal for help, or for release from this obsessive ailment of the astral existence.

Perhaps the best solution lies in obtaining the help of a psychic sensitive, and not a charlatan ghost catcher, so popular with the lower social strata of psychic ignorance. The methods of telepathic communication with understanding of the hypothesis which I have advanced, even in the form of sincere prayer, directed with the sole purpose to help to relieve the obsession might be successful.

I base these conclusions on numerous letters which unwittingly convey the information that when people became interested, and understood that their thoughts could perhaps be helpful, and that the haunts were motivated by some sort of need; this attitude of mind, this reliance on their thoughts to help, often brought about cessation of the phenomena. As in the case of the blind old man, telepathy cannot be underestimated in these cases.

From Mr. Sadie's collection I wish to relate this amazing re-enactment of a tragedy as told by Mrs. J. A. van Blerk of Geluk in the district of Brits. She relates in Afrikaans :

"It was in 1910. My father had sold his farm and we rented a house on the outskirts of Vryheid. The house was on a plot fronted by a row of bluegum trees next to the fence.

"One September evening my father was not at home and my mother and my elder sister were in the diningroom. We had finished supper so my younger sister and I went to the sittingroom. She began to play the piano and I stood next to her facing the front door which was open. While standing there listening to her playing I saw someone throw a burning cigar stump up against the verandah so that the sparks went flying in several directions.

"I thought it was a guest, and went to the door but there was no one. While I was standing on the stoep looking for this person who had thrown the cigar stump, I noticed a man dressed in a grey raincoat and white trousers coming towards the stoep from the gate. He had a cloth cap on his head, but I could not see his face distinctly, he was however smoking a cigar and I could see the red glow of the cigar in the dusk of the evening.

"I watched him and as he reached the stoep he stopped and threw the burning cigar against the verandah roof and again the sparks flew in all directions. I could see he was a white man as he came up to me. I first addressed him in Afrikaans, and when he did not answer me I spoke in English, but it appeared as if he just did not understand what I was saying. I wondered whether I had perhaps not made a mistake, and that he might not be a white man, so I spoke to him in a Bantu language.

"This I should not have done. He lifted his hand to smack my face, and I jumped back as quickly as I could but he was like lightning and smacked me on my cheek. It was exactly as if I were struck against the head by an air-cushion. When I looked again he was gone. I went indoors, naturally upset and told my mother and my sisters what had happened.

"A little later my mother was standing looking out of the window; she saw the dogs barking furiously and snarl as if something terrible was upsetting them. My mother then called us to come and witness what strange happening was taking place. When I reached the window I saw a huge wagon loaded high standing under the bluegum trees not far from the house. At once six natives arrived who began to unload the stuff from the wagon, and I could distinctly see rolls of linen. The dogs with hair raised up on their backs were leaping up, snapping, barking and snarling, but keeping well away from the wagon and the natives.

Then all at once the natives were gone, and we saw two white policemen and a native policeman who began to load the goods back on to the wagon. Then we saw them pick up a stretcher with someone lying on it. They carried the person away. Suddenly there was no wagon, and the dogs stopped barking and just walked around normally.

But of course we were nonplussed and wondered what it all

meant when while still at the window watching this scene of unnatural activity, we saw the same man coming up to the stoep, and again he took the glowing cigar, and threw it against the house. The moment he had done this the wagon reappeared under the trees, and the natives were unloading it exactly as they had done a few minutes before. This performance as we had seen it from the beginning, was repeated over and over again until about 3 a.m., when all suddenly stopped, the dogs gave up their vigil and their barking and went to sleep.

As soon as it was daylight we went to investigate and as there had been a soft misty rain that night we expected if the happenings had been real to find impressions of wagon wheels and human tracks. But we found nothing of the sort. The next morning we spoke to a neighbour a Mr. van Rensburg about our strange visions of the night before. He then told us something which none of us had heard, and of which we had no knowledge whatsoever.

He described how a Scotch trader with his wagon of goods, which served as his shop, traded all over the district, especially with the natives. But whenever he came to town he always outspanned on the same spot under the buegum trees on the property which we were occupying, because the people who lived in the house at that time were great friends of his.

Then one misty rainy night in September 1907 he again outspanned in his usual place under the bluegum trees. During that night he was attacked and murdered by natives, and his wagon plundered. The police found him the next morning dead, dressed in a grey raincoat and white trousers and he still had a cap on his head. What was portrayed repeatedly that night fitted the account of his murder, and the stealing of the goods, which we witnessed as a ghostly scene."

This is an extremely interesting and authentic description of a ghost scene, but there are some components of the events as perceived by Mrs. van Blerk and her family which require analysis. We learn that the Scotsman outspanned on the property of his friends. Therefore if there were people in the house that night they might have been able to hear his call for help if he did so. Furthermore it is unlikely that if there were people sleeping nearby that the natives would have taken their time in unloading the goods, including rolls of linen. Again, if he had come to the house for help as Mrs. van Blerk saw him, he would hardly have adopted an aggressive and annoyed attitude by throwing his cigar against the house. His attitude towards Mrs. van Blerk, when he smacked her, indicated that he was not wounded and in need of help.

If all the items of the haunt belonged faithfully to a past memory and were reproduced as such, then one should ask why there was no female on the stoep whom he smacked in the scenes which were witnessed from the window? Again it is most improbable that a man who outspanned on his friend's property should have been in the habit of coming up to his house and throwing his glowing cigar against his verandah or front wall.

These items seem somehow not to be appropriate to the relationship of this man to the family who lived there, nor to the circumstances of his murder. They seem to suggest anger, annoyance and an attempt to draw attention to something on his mind, something which obsessed his thoughts, and bound him to that locality.

He was dissatisfied and angry. Let us interpret the picture in accordance with the nature of the behaviour of the discarnate Scotsman. It is known that this trader was murdered at his wagon by natives on a misty rainy night near the house of his friends. But it is not known whether the people were at home that night, nor whether the murderers were ever caught and punished.

The police came and took his body away on a stretcher, and even loaded the scattered goods found on the ground back on to the wagon. All that the scene portrayed was firstly the man coming up to the house with a glowing cigar and then flinging it with anger against the front of the house. Thereafter the scene at the wagon followed. There was no presentation as to the manner of his death; all that was presented to the astral vision of those at the window was the unloading of the goods by about six natives; then this scene faded and was followed by the police loading the goods on to the wagon and carrying the body away on a stretcher.

It seems therefore more in keeping with the events to accept that the trader on the astral after his death had not accepted his transition. He was still enslaved by the thoughts that he had been robbed by natives, and that these robbers had not been brought to book. The absence of the scene of his death strongly indicates that he was under the impression that he was still on the earth, and that he wanted justice done. He was not aware that he had died. Hence the death-scene or the actual murder was not part of the memory which he projected and re-enacted on the astral plane.

I consider that the absence of the scene of his actual murder was most significant and showed that the drama witnessed by Mrs. van Blerk and her family members was a mental picture, as well as the state of mind of the earthbound discarnate Scotch trader. It did not appear as an impression made on so-called ether, which was mechanically re-enacted without any thinker, or any dynamic factor of a living psyche employing memories to express a dissatisfied mind. The ghostly scene witnessed by the women at the window was apparently that part of his memories which formed a general impression of what had happened that misty rainy night.

But we cannot avoid seeing him in this particular scene with Mrs. van Blerk as essentially an actor adapting himself to new circumstances. For example, when she addressed him after he had thrown his cigar in anger against the wall or verandah she asked him what she could do for him. First she spoke in Afrikaans, then in English, and when he made no response, she addressed him in a Bantu language. His immediate reaction to this language clearly indicated a resentment relative to that particular moment. It could not have been part of the original murder and its associations, because there is no evidence that there had been a woman on the stoep on the night of the murder. Besides if there were such a person the events would have been different and Mr. van Rensburg's account of the murder would have been different. The anger and the smacking on the face of Mrs. van Blerk were reactions to new circumstances.

The murdered trader did not know that his astral existence was a process which followed death. The witnesses never saw him being murdered in the repeated ghost scene. If he had known that he was dead the murder-scene might have been re-enacted. But the impression is that he was concerned with the robbery of his goods. His preoccupation on the astral was with his trading and the catching of the thieves and other grievances related to that night. Perhaps on the night of the murder he had gone to the house for assistance and found no one at home. He must have slept at his wagon to guard his goods.

We can now picture a misty rainy night with coincidence of astral memories and the earthly scene, and several females in a house all possessing some degree of psycnic power, thus setting up a magnetic field with their auras. Our astral trader, not knowing that he had died was drawn to this scene of his grievances and the wrongs which he had suffered at the hands of the natives. Perhaps Mrs. van Blerk was not clairaudient and so could not hear astrally what he said. He could have been speaking all the time but her astral inability to receive his communication could have incensed him still further until, when addressed in a Bantu language he had lost his temper completely.

The omission from the psychic scene of his actual murder is of great significance and to my mind is a repressed memory or amnesia because he had no insight into his real mind. He did not realize that he had been murdered. We might ask why then did the astral memories present the police with the body on a stretcher? This could of course be part of the general impression without his knowing that the body was dead, because at that time he was possessed by the thoughts of loss and the robbery.

The dogs were indeed reliable witnesses. They saw with their astral sight the scene enacted on the astral dimensionality but coinciding with that locality. In consequence they did not bark and snarl at a thought but at substantial beings and objects at the wagon. As soon as the picture seen by the women disappeared the dogs were quiet, and walked about calmly, but the moment the women saw the beginning of this astral drama, the dogs would close in towards the wagon barking fiercely but never approaching too near to the wagon.

This synchronising of perception between the women and the dogs does show that the scene was an independent portrayal, happening in a substantial medium of energy on the astral plane. On that particular night a series of factors came together to open the album of eternity. Another world of vibrations with a dynamic astral agent had intruded on an earthly night with the women and the dogs as the audience.

Mrs. Pamela Yates told me about an experience with their female spaniel. They were living in a new house at Amsterdam Hoek near Port Elizabeth. They noticed that at times the dog would look at something on the same level as its head, not up or down, but staring in front of her at something which they could not see. After a few moments she would whimper with terror and even on occasions almost foamed at the mouth. Then in a terror-stricken state she would leap onto Mr. Yates' bed and scratch furiously to get under the bedclothes where she would crawl next to him shaking and trembling.

They carefully observed this unexplained and apparently causeless behaviour of the dog, trying to find an explanation for it. There were occasions when she would sit and watch the door and then just stare straight in front of her with her hair standing on end; then she would yelp and flee for protection. Mrs. Yates and her husband came to the conclusion that the phantom of some frightening creature stalked her and was only seen by her, causing her to whimper and seek human protection. It could have been the phantom of another vicious dog—an astral visitor like the trader and his cigar? But other people who love animals have observed doggie behaviour which is worth mentioning.

One particular case was brought to my notice by a lady. She had two little terriers and one died. For some days the other one would hardly eat and seemed definitely sad. Now these two used to chase each other round the house from room to room, scattering the small rugs. They used to lie with their front legs down looking at each other and then suddenly dart off in a wild scamper.

One morning she was on top of the stairs looking down into the hall where her doggie was lying. Then she saw him slowly raise himself and wag his tail. His back was towards her. He pulled his ears back, as he used to do when happy and playful. And then he went down on his front legs, wagged his tail and darted off in a wild scamper. Then he stopped and looked surprised. But thereafter she observed this game on several occasions. She wanted to know whether his little pal had come back to play with him? At that time I thought there might have been another explanation. But since then I have heard of several similar observations of doggie behaviour.

When we think of the behaviour of the dogs when Mrs. van Blerk witnessed the ghost-scene near the wagon, then there is no reason not to accept the possibility of an astral doggie visiting his old home and his pals and perhaps even playing with them. The world of haunts is a world with phenomena which arise from emotion and thought pressing in certain directions and operating on energy systems as yet far beyond our rational knowledge. Somehow the field of force conception which we radiate seem to provide the best approach to this deeper understanding.

The late General Smuts was a man who vibrated so intimately with the forces of nature, that he could not fail to feel the reality of this concept. Some years after I had begun to believe in this human magnetic field of force, mainly as a result of the trumpet and the reactions of the Scotch medium, I read *Holism and Evolution* by J. C. Smuts. He wrote :

"Things, ideas, animals, plants, persons : all these, like physical forces, have their fields, and but for their fields they would be unintelligible, their activities would be impossible, and their relations barren and sterile."

CHAPTER V

PHANTOMS, VISIONS AND PREMONITIONS

Mr. C. of Stilfontein wrote to me in Afrikaans that since his early childhood he has been clairvoyant and seen visions. Telepathic experiences were quite common and so were premonitions. All these phenomena he accepted as part of his daily life. He found however that as he grew older these supernormal perceptions became less and less clear.

He had been reared in a religious churchianic home. His father had been a minister of the Dutch Reformed Church. During 1934 his father had died, and in the absence of the disciplinary influence exercised by his father during his life-time Mr. C became wayward. He mixed with people not of his class, and began to drink at a very early age. His mother was shocked and felt quite at a loss as to what to do. He was devil-may-care, and as a teenager would often come home under the influence of alcohol.

Then one evening he came home intoxicated and threw himself on his bed. But he could not sleep; a strange wakefulness possessed him, so he lay there on his back staring at the ceiling, waiting for what he knew not. And then he saw his deceased father next to his bed—he had on his toga, but his expression was furious. He raised his right fist in his direction. He approached the bed with eyes glowing like coals of fire.

This terrific display of anger by his father paralysed him with fear. He could feel the cold perspiration streaming down his body. He was definitely not asleep for he could hear all the night noises and the roar of the waves. They were at the seaside. He could hear the crickets and the noise in the street of the holidaymakers; all these during the moments when his father stood there in that mood. His little dog which slept in his room gave one howl and ran away.

His father came slowly nearer until he was bending over him and he could feel a warm radiation from the phantom figure. Then all at once his father pressed his left palm with fingers spread out firmly on his chest. He smiled and just disappeared. A cool air surrounded him and his fear went—in the room was a scent, sweet and refreshing.

Mr. C. was fifteen years old at the time of this experience but the marks of the five fingers remained on his chest, and whenever he was in a temper then the marks of the fingers became more distinct, as though the blood vessels dilated in that area. Gradually in the course of the years these impressions faded. He however never touched alcohol again, and became determined never to relapse.

Mr. C went on to describe how he grew up at Somerset Strand. One Sunday afternoon at Melkbaai he was lying sunbathing some distance from the sea, on the sand when all of a sudden he saw right in front of his eyes a lovely little blonde girl of about five-years old. She had on a little red bathing costume and he distinctly heard her say "Uncle (oom) please help me, I am drowning."

He jumped up from where he was lying and ran towards the sea, and as he reached the water he saw a little figure bobbing up and down in the waves, with blonde hair and a little red bathing costume showing on the water. She was blue in the face already. He rendered first-aid and artificial respiration, and as she had not inspired much water she was soon well and crying loudly. He handed this unknown child to its shocked mother.

He continued :

"I had a friend in Krugersdorp who was a drunkard. His wife and children had to suffer in consequence. This was a great pity as he had a good background and came from an educated family. My wife and I rented a little house on his plot. Then one bright moonlight night his mother appeared to me. I never knew the little old lady during her life-time. My friend never talked to me about his parents and I had not seen a photograph of them in his house.

This apparition of a delicate old lady appeared to me in a black Boer "kappie" and a black dress, and sat near the back door on the wall of our fishpond. I could see in the depth of the "kappie" a very attractive face staring at me with great sadness of the eyes. On her left temple was a large and distinct mole. She spoke to me telepathically but I could hear her words as if spoken deep within me :— "Tell my son I have no rest, and can't find the happiness in store for me because of his excessive drinking and its effects on his family."

Having spoken she disappeared. I saw her son and told him of my experience and the outstanding characteristics of the person I had never seen in physical form. He was very surprised and thereafter made a serious attempt to control his drinking. Some months later when his efforts were definitely bearing fruit and his drinking habits had changed for the better, she again appeared, in my bedroom, but this time she smiled sweetly and seemed very happy. I never saw her again."

Mr. C. mentioned several other similar experiences where phantoms warned him of accidents. These premonitions always took the form of the appearance of a phantom. His clairvoyant faculty was of course well developed. The apparitions were, according to his evidence, those of discarnate beings. His father came to show his intense displeasure at his son's conduct, and then with a highly condensed and concentrated energy of an astral hand left an impression of five fingers on his chest.

This episode reminds one of Genesis IV verse 15 :— "And the Lord set a mark upon Cain, lest any finding him should kill him." The incident of the little blonde girl in the red bathing costume is difficult to explain, except by means of automatic projection of her astral body. As the child became unconscious the astral separated and was then evidently drawn to the field of force of Mr. C. Being psychic he was easily contacted by her astral personality.

Here then the astral was seeking help for its physical body, and in so doing appeared distinctly to Mr. C.'s astral sight; although he could not see the sea, or the little girl from where he was lying. The instinct for self-preservation could therefore be active even in the astral consciousness.

An ex-officer of the Indian Army who wished to remain anonymous wrote to me of an occasion of a dinner party in India. Towards the end of the dinner Major T. suddenly jumped up from the table and said :— "My mother is dead," and pointing to some Arum lilies in a vase in the centre of the table, said :— "I can see her in that lily. She is lying in her bed dead."

Then he staggered from the room—got into his trap and drove away. They thought that perhaps Major T. had had a little too much to drink but were reassured on that point when a cablegram arrived from England giving the mother's death at the time when he saw her in the lily."

Now who was responsible for this perception? Did Major T. see his mother clairvoyantly without any intention from her side? I do not think so. I think the idea was initiated by his mother the moment she found herself on the astral plane. Her idea was to convey the impression to him that she had passed over, and since Arum lilies are frequently associated with death she chose this flower to project a thoughtform of herself as she was lying in her bed.

The astral plane is evidently the plane for manifestation of thoughtforms which seem to take on a substantial appearance because of this particular energy system. In the same way would I consider that thoughtforms entering someone's aura or field of force could at times absorb sufficient energy so as to become substantial as a phantasm.

A lady wrote to tell me how, while on a visit in the South of England she bought herself a new mauve dress for a party. Her husband and the children were at home a few hundred miles away. After she had dressed herself and felt quite pleased with her attractive appearance in her smart mauve dress, she wished that her husband could see her at that moment to see how smart and well she looked. At that time the husband at home looked up from reading his paper to find his wife standing in front of him looking radiant in her new mauve dress. When notes were compared afterwards there was no doubt that he had seen a substantial phantasm of his wife as she wanted him to see her.

Here then I think the thoughtform was transmitted telepathically but took substance for its manifestation from the aura of her husband. It has always seemed to me that even tunes which sometimes persist in running through one's head could be caught up within the field of force of one's aura.

The phantom companions which the magicians in Tibet made for themselves, as experienced by Mrs. Alexandra David Neel, could not have assumed the substantial forms which they did if it were not for the aura which was triggered by thoughtforms which themselves possessed the properties of a magnetic nature.

In an interesting letter Mrs. May Davies from Pinelands in the Cape told of the following experience :— "Sunday January the 8th 1961 was the usual kind of Sunday in my household; a casual breakfast, a quick glance at the paper and then gathering together the ingredients that go towards making a picnic a success."

Mrs. Davies suffered from migraine. "Quite suddenly while packing the basket I developed a blinding headache, and an ache in all my limbs that was unbearable. I reached out for my husband's arm for I was blinded with pain. "I can't go out today. I must lie down, please let me stay in the dark and please put some ice on my head."

My husband did all these things and I lay not on the bed but on the settee in the lounge, where I could feel the wind on my face and get the sea smell. This was strange because with such a headache I usually only wanted the quiet and the dark. I lay, sometimes saying "Please God take this pain away," or just lay waiting for the waves of nausea to go, resentful and disappointed because my Sunday had been spoiled.

Then suddenly my mother came and stood by the settee. She looked many years younger than when I had last visited her in England five years before. "I have come to have a look at your view before I die, and to see you then I can die happy," she said. I got up from the settee, took her hand and said :— "Don't be silly Mom, you are not going to die." She folded her hands in her apron, a trick she had of doing when talking. It was an apron made of hessian and I remembered how she used to wear it over her skirt when she scrubbed the kitchen floor when I was a little girl.

"Come on our May," she said, "show me the view from the verandah that you are always writing 'ome about." We went on to the stoep together and looked at the sea sparkling silvery white with waves. We looked at the view across from Mouille Point towards Blaauwberg Strand and the mountains beyond. My Mom sighed. "Don't it smell nice," she said. Then turning to me she smiled. "I am so glad I've seen it, now I can die 'appy."

We both stepped back from the stoep into the lounge. My Mom walked a few steps with me, smiled and was gone. I was not lying on the settee any more, but standing in the room when I came to. I did not feel afraid; she had been so real and not ghost-like. I went through the flat into the kitchen where my husband was making a cup of tea. "Did you hear me talking?" I asked. "Not a word." I tried again. "My Mom has been to see me. I think she is ill. I think she is going to die."

My husband did not laugh. "It could be my girl," he said. "And if your Mom is passing on, you are the first one she will try to tell." Well we drank tea, I cried a great deal because England and my Mom were so far away. Then I wandered through the lounge hoping to see her again, but there was no one there. I must have dreamed it, I thought. On the Tuesday evening January 10th, the cablegram arrived dated January 10th, 8 a.m. "Mom passed away early today—cremation date later. From Dad."

Mrs. Davies has had other clairvoyant visions of a lady who once lived in a house in Boksburg. She is therefore a psychic sensitive with good astral vision for this world. It appears that her attack of migraine passed over during the interview with her mother. The interesting factor in this whole experience is whether her mother was a mere projected thoughtform brought about by her desire to see her daughter, knowing that her time was near, or was it an astral projection which happened in the same manner but which required sleep, unconsciousness or deep exhaustion from illness, where the person is not trained to perform a voluntary feat of this nature.

The degree of animation, the interest, the familiar characteristics and the domestic dress as I shall call her little apron were all added to fill out the picture of recognition and to produce the known personality. In any case Mrs. Davies' psychic constitution created the conditions of energy by means of which her mother could take on a definite astral form and converse in a manner which meant to inform her daughter of her coming departure from earth life.

It is most probable that this was a visit on the astral plane and not the physical world of sense perception. The vision of Mrs. Davies was astral and her conversation was astral hence her husband, a few yards away, never heard a word. It can be surmised that her mother at the time of her projection and appearance to her daughter was probably unconscious.

A few years ago Mrs. Shearer's mother was seriously ill in hospital. Her daughter with her grandchildren were down on holiday in Port Elizabeth. The serious illness of their "greatgrannie" was not told them and the impression was created that she would get well and come home after the operation. There was always a member of the family with her during the later period when she became comatosed. Anyway the grandchildren knew none of this.

Then one afternoon the little grandson aged five was playing outside the kitchen door in the back garden. Mrs. Shearer, his mother, a Miss Pretorius and a coloured servant were all in the kitchen when he came in hurriedly from his game, as if he had been interrupted in his play. As he came in he said to them :— "I have just seen 'greatgrannie' going up, up there in the sky. She was going to heaven." They were amazed and Mrs. Shearer questioned him about her appearance, dress and so on, and he answered most unconcernedly as if he were describing an everyday occurrence, "Oh she was dressed in white and she was going up and up over there," pointing to the sky and then he went out to continue his game. Within moments of this conversation, in fact they were still looking at each other in astonishment, the 'phone rang and her brother told her that their mother had died a few minutes before.

Here then was a little boy playing at a game and suddenly he saw a vision of his "greatgrannie" who died at a time of which he had no other source of knowledge. The realities of the situation are such that one must conclude that he had an astral vision of his "greatgrannie" and that she telepathically drew his attention to her departure. It is somewhat significant that the grandson of a mediumistic person should show these extrasensory faculties, which do indicate that these constitutional factors could have a hereditary basis.

Mrs. C. du Plessis wrote to me about the only occasion in her life when she saw a vision of light. "I woke early in the morning to feel whether my sick baby whom I had taken into bed with me was still covered. As I did so my attention was drawn to a small light, resembling a little sun. It moved several times : I thought three. It moved up and down and then disappeared. The night was very dark and there was no moon. Within three months of the appearance of the light I lost my baby; my sister and sister-in-law each lost a child. I associate the three deaths with the three movements of the light.

I have numerous letters in Afrikaans mentioning premonitions of death which were symbolised by a light, usually a ball of light. It is believed that these are ectoplasmic manifestations manipulated by discarnate relatives or friends. I have often wondered whether these almost substantial manifestations were not somehow part of the instinct of self-preservation forming in a manner a subconscious link with those beyond by means of astral feeling and knowing? It could be that at certain appropriate moments, when the power is of sufficient intensity from this side, that these phenomena make their appearance in the nature of the materialization of thought, usually in a symbolic form.

Mrs. K. the mother of a friend of mine had never had any psychic experiences, and perhaps never gave these matters any thought. She had a bosom friend, a Mrs. Bosch who had died some months before. One morning Mrs. K. was having tea with some friends, and in the middle of their conversation she exclaimed, pointing at the door :— "Good heavens, look there stands my friend Mrs. Bosch and she is waving to me and smiling so happily." A few days later Mrs K. died of a stroke.

The reasonable conclusion is that Mrs. Bosch, knowing that her friend was going to die found that moment with a number of people together the most suitable time to make her astral appearance, and to impress on her friend, that she was still very much alive. Who knows but that there could have been some unconscious medium in that group, who provided the major portion of the field of force for Mrs. Bosch to become astrally visible to Mrs. K. It could also have been a projection of a thoughtform by Mrs. Bosch, which assumed astral visibility because of the field of force produced in the room. The operation of these laws offers a promise of a far-reaching science of the future and perhaps of a higher humanity.

A Mr. S. sent me an interesting story which was vouched for by several most respected burghers and happened between 1880 and 1890. His father and several friends came by wagon from Sutherland to Ceres. They outspanned in the veld and prepared supper. While they were eating around the camp-fire miles from nowhere, a huge black dog appeared amongst them. One of the men was just going to stroke this lovely dog, when his father told this man not to do so as it was not a physical dog. The moment he said this the dog just disappeared from their midst. It just melted into nothing.

No one had any misfortune and no one associated this dog with some ill-omen. In view of the phenomena for which astral manifestation can be held responsible I would venture to speculate that this dog had been lost in the wilds from the wagon of some trekker. That evening when the familiar scene was reflected on the astral plane, his past memories of his search for his master actuated him, and making use of the field of force provided by the personalities present he did what he had done so often before, and mixed freely with the group around the camp-fire near the wagon. The fact that he was seen by all present showed that the persons shared a fair faculty for astral vision.

Mr. P. of the Calvinia district described an experience in which the actions of a phantom of his deceased sister-in-law conveyed their meaning clearly to him and determined his decision. He wrote :— "It was about fifteen years ago when my sister-in-law died and left two small children, both little girls. Three days after the funeral I was just getting into bed for my night's rest—the light was still burning, when there came into the room my deceased sister-in-law with a child in each arm. She never spoke a word. There was not a sound but she stood there as she had been in life, and all she did was to hold out the two little girls towards me. Then she turned round and went out of the door with the children on her arms.

I decided that she wanted me to adopt the children which I did the next day. They are two happy girls at school today, the one seventeen and the other fifteen years old. This was no imagination or hallucination—the person was substantial with features clearly distinct." He accepted that she appeared from the other world to place her children in his care. This picture connotes that the mother, after her death became concerned about the welfare of her children left behind. She therefore produced a distinct thoughtform of herself and her children; phantasms of three beings, and by symbolic gesture made her meaning perfectly clear.

Here again I consider that Mr. P. at that moment radiated sufficient energy for this manifestation to become so life-like. But the lesson of this apparition is the role of the departed mother, and her appearance as an active agent concerned with the future of her children. If there is no survival of an astral personality, who could have been responsible for this directive of thought, this maternal concern, and the dramatic appeal of the phantom's outstretched arms? The only person who could have served as a cause for such a portrayal was the deceased mother.

Mr. C. Rubidge of Richmond in the Cape Province wrote as follows :—"The farm I am on belonged at one time to the late President Burgers. I took over in 1924 and I might mention that I had never been in this part of the country before. I had to work hard and had no difficulty in falling asleep, but great difficulty in waking up.

Then one night we had visitors, but unfortunately one of our children was not well and so my wife and the sick child slept in one room and I with the baby in another. The next morning I woke early and was immediately conscious of a presence in the room and I could dimly discern a shape. There, levitated about a foot away from the foot-end of the bed was a woman with her hair rolled up in a bun and wearing a tulle dress. She resembled my mother. She came near and stroked my little girl. I had no sense of fear, but felt that I wanted to protect my little girl and at the same time I pinched myself to make quite sure that I was awake.

The face of the apparition was not turned towards me. Her movements were like those which one sees in a slow-motion picture. Then she turned away and disappeared towards the corner of the room. We were interested in the phenomenon and made inquiries. We learned of an old lady who had died in the house and who always wore brown—just as I saw on the apparition. Every detail which I saw was verified by people who had known her; in particular her fondness for brown dresses and her tremendous affection for children. She had lost a little two-year old daughter; the age of my little girl whom she came to stroke so gently."

It was authentically established that a lady of that appearance and characteristics had lived in that house, and that her little girl of two years had died there. This visit by a discarnate form was not in any way a premonition, nor was the person, during her life-time on earth known to Mr. Rubidge and his family. Hence one must conclude that this appearance from out of the blue which never recurred again, was a conscious intention of an astral being who knew the place and who probably on visiting it because of memories, saw the little girl who reminded her of her own, and as there was power for the purpose she became visible in astral form.

There was no wish from this side of the grave for her to appear except her own desires and her own mental intentions and satisfactions. From this experience one can draw the conclusion that discarnate beings can go visiting on their own will and desires. Maybe she had a function on the other side, which concerned little children—some sort of foster mother perhaps.

Mr. W. wrote from the Eastern Transvaal about the curious behaviour of a ghost.

"About three years ago a very old friend of ours died. He was seventy-eight and rather a lonely character. During the last three or four months of his life, he used to visit us on our farm at least three times a week. He always came at tea times and always wore the same light-grey suit. He had a very prominent nose.

"We had a youngish friend, a woman who had just lost her husband staying with us, and she slept in an outside room. Our old friend Archie, a naughty old man, always followed the same procedure on his visits. He would get out of his car and would walk straight past the house to our friend's bedroom. There he would press his face against the window pane and peer in for a minute or more, and if no one was in the room, he would then come to the stoep for tea.

"In four months he must have done this about fifty times. He was quite blatant about it even if a few of us were watching him from the stoep, he'd still peer through that window before joining us. Shortly after his death, our woman friend returned to her home, and a couple from Zululand came to spend a week with us. They occupied the room which she had stayed in. They arrived about 3.30 p.m. and after a bath and change came on to the stoep for tea."

Then her husband said :

"'Who's the old chap who looked through the window when Joan (his wife) was dressing?'" We assured him that no one had been near, and he then described our old friend Archie : grey suit, rather scruffy-looking and prominent nose. He never appeared again. Joan is rather given to seeing things whereas her husband is completely materialistic. This is utterly and absolutely authentic."

Unfortunately Mr. W. did not mention whether Joan or her husband saw the figure of Archie. If Joan were known to be psychically sensitive then it meant that she provided the power for Archie to be seen and also no doubt attracted his dominating earthly curiosity about women. The repetition of a state of mind which he indulged in during earth life perhaps actuated by phantasy and desires for the young widow, was repeated by him but strangely enough only once. In spite of the fact that Joan was psychic, they never saw him again.

If he were dominated by an earth-bound impulse and if his deed were a spiritless photograph of his previous habit, he should not have vanished for good once he saw that the woman in the room was not the young widow. The cessation of his visits even in astral form, does suggest that he realized she was not the person he was interested in, and hence show the operation of will and choice of a surviving personality.

Mrs. D. writing from Durban says :

"I can honestly tell you that I have a familiar 'something' which has made itself known to me in the shape of a black Scotch terrier dog. This being was seen by me many times, usually when something was about to happen to me personally, but not always in connection with misfortune. It appears at my side as if following me.

"The first time I experienced its presence was when I was

dressing to go out, and as I came from the bathroom into the bedroom I saw this black dog at my side. I looked at it for some minutes thinking it was a strange dog that had invaded the house, so I went to the door and called my daughter to take him out. But as I turned back to the room he was gone. This happened several years ago but I still have him with me. Now before you exclaim in disbelief let me assure you that I do not drink, nor suffer from nerves, or hallucinations, nor am I over-imaginative."

Several people have written about seeing animals, mostly dogs. I don't think Mrs. D. meant by "familiar" the ancient idea of a spirit which is supposed to obey and attend a sorcerer. If we assume that the next stage of life after death is one in an astral dimensionality, then there is no reason why dogs and cats and other domesticated animals should not in astral form be actuated by previous memories and associations.

We have no knowledge what laws or vibrations determine such associations as mentioned by Mrs. D. but although supernormal the association could still be quite natural. The astral doggie had found a companion, something about Mrs. D. had attracted him, and since his advent to her home he has acted as her guardian and has appeared on certain significant occasions. We of course do not know whether he is also not associated with someone else on the astral who employs the doggie for the purpose of making Mrs. D. aware of certain events. There need not be anything sinister in these phenomena.

Mr. S. writing from the Pretoria district described a peculiar light that appeared in a certain locality. It would travel along the road parallel with a car. Often it would suddenly appear and hover about for a while and then disappear. Numerous people have seen it. It always started from a certain patch of thorn trees.

He heard from his grandfather that at the beginning of this century he had come upon a corpse in a state of decomposition underneath those thick thorn trees. It was that of a white person clad in a brown suit and brown shoes and believed to be that of an Englishman. The body had been buried there under the thorn trees where it had been found, and it has been since that time that a light has haunted the area.

Visions of lights as haunts are very common in South Africa judging by the number of letters on this subject which came to hand. Now lights are manifestations often seen in the presence of physical mediums and those who produce ectoplasm. It is therefore a phenomenon which is associated with the presence of discarante beings or their influence. Many people think they are forms of ectoplasmic glowing. It could be that for some reason or other the person buried under the thorn trees wanted to draw attention to his grave and identity. Often there are ideas which must be expressed, because of their pressing importance to the person.

If then these ideas continued to operate on the astral and concerned others living in this world, the symbol of light could be used to help find a solution to his problem. Man's primitive reactions which place sinister interpretations on visions of this nature might often prevent people from solving some mystery.

Mr. Sp. writing from Pietermaritzburg told about his unique experience as follows :

"It was a bright sunny day in May 1938 in Pietermaritzburg. My wife and I who were in this city on holiday were walking along one of the main thoroughfares in a residential area, when we entered a narrow street on our way to friends. This was practically a lane; I noticed that a car was parked on one side facing towards me, and that a little group of people were going down this street. We were walking briskly and soon caught up with this group which consisted of a little old woman, dressed all in black, and a few paces behind her were four boys from fourteen to fifteen years of age.

"I did not notice anything about the woman's costume to date it, but I was surprised to see that the boys were dressed in a style which had been common during the early years of the century, but which had gone out of fashion since the 1914-1918 war. These boys, although barefooted all wore blue peaked caps, blue polo-necked jerseys and rather long shorts. They had a poverty-stricken appearance and the fact that they were shoeless on a cold day confirmed this. I also wondered why they were not at school. As we passed them I was shocked to hear that they were baiting the old woman, passing such rude remarks as 'Go on you old witch' and 'You are a witch.'

"The poor old woman looked dreadfully harassed and as we passed she entered the front gate of one of the houses. The boys stood in a group in front of the gate and continued to call out to her. Now in the ordinary way I would have choked them off as hooligans but while I wanted to do this something within me prevented me. I seemed to realize somehow that I could do nothing to protect the old woman from her tormentors. As we passed I turned to my wife and asked her whether she did not agree that what we had just witnessed was disgraceful.

"She looked at me with amazement all over her face and said that she did not know what I was talking about. I started to explain but her amazement grew, and as I turned round to show her the group of boys the street was deserted. It was impossible for boys to have run away in that short time. I am completely at a loss to account for this event. I am not psychic and this is the only experience of this kind that I have ever had." Mrs. Sp. added her recollections of what her husband had told her on that occasion.

This type of experience is called retrocognition, which means knowledge acquired of some past event other than by means of the senses. In reality it is knowledge not inferred from any suggestion or sense impression, but seems to come from beyond the range of a person's memory. The famous "Petit Trianon" case, which was experienced and described by Miss Moberley who was then principal of St. Hugh's College, Oxford, and Miss Jourdain the vice-principal, is a typical example. These two ladies in August 1901, when visiting the Petit Trianon at Versailles, saw a scene in the time of Marie Antoinette, which must have happened more than a century before the time these ladies perceived it.

It was a live scene in which several persons took part. It was vivid in broad daylight. The information gathered from that vision was afterwards confirmed by documents in the French National Archives. The experience is described in a book called "An Adventure" by Anne Moberley and Eleanor Jourdain.

There are many other accounts of retrocognition on record; several complex, if not perplexing explanations have been advanced, which often just become lost in words. I think that since there is abundant evidence of an astral dimensionality and even a body of an inner personality one must seek the explanation for these phenomena on that plane.

From time immemorial man has made some reference to universal recording of our earthly happenings. Man's religious conception of a Judgment Day refers to some recording of memories of one's deeds. Then there is for example the Jewish greeting during their New Year, when Jewish people greet each other with the holiday formula : "leshanah tobah Tikkateb" meaning "May you be written down in the book of life for a good year." This ancient conception therefore of recording man's actions and deeds, is a symbolic way of describing an intuitive conception of some universal or world memory.

There must have been somewhere in man's past psychic life experiences of the same nature as retrocognition of today, as well as precognition of events, which had not taken place on earth at the time, and we can infer that from these psychic phenomena, especially retrocognition man derived the idea of a book of life in which happenings and deeds were recorded. The book idea is a mere personification of God as an eternal recorder of our actions, and fitted in with a religion based primarily on the wrath of a personal God, who would ultimately meet out justice as we find in "The Egyptian Book of the Dead."

Nowadays these scenes of a past age or even more remote periods, which are seen by people, are ascribed to a persistent memory in what is known as the psychic ether. Others suggest that the observer might have been influenced telepathically by the discarnate being who saw the scene during his life on earth. I am more inclined to take cognisance of the ancient conception of a record of the earth's happenings, where it affected the minds of man, and that these were in existence on some plane in the cosmos.

In the first place we only know memory as part of our physical existence; that is, receiving impressions, retaining them and recalling them when necessary, but what memory is in itself outside our brains we have no idea. Hence in following the clue of ancient thought, I am disposed to consider the astral dimensionality or plane as it is also called, as the first plane where the memories of the earth are retained. They are carried over by minds from the earth, and are probably somehow recorded there by means beyond our comprehension.

I have advanced the idea that there is some reflection and correspondence on the densest portions of the astral of the topography of this earth; the same as the reflection in the water of banks and trees on the side of a river. With this exception, that on the astral these are substantial because they are formed out of astral energy as part of the energy spectrum of the cosmos.

Hence a scene of human activity with its emotional elements must become part of the memories of those who figured in it, and as these memories are taken along after death to the first or next plane of our existence, some record of them must remain there, as long as currents of thoughts, memories and images have dynamic power and magnetise the astral atmospheres.

Let us assume on this hypothesis, as I have mentioned before but which is worth repeating in the case of retrocognition, that there is a law which at times brings the astral reflections, resemblances or localities and their memories into coincidence with the material earth; as a hand fits into a glove. Should this happen and the memories are still part of discarnate minds on the astral plane, then a psychic sensitive, with an increased power of astral sight in the physical observer, could behold the scene and its characters of the past as happening there and then. This is what I think happened to Mr. Sp. on that May day in Pietermaritzburg.

Let us look at the following dramatic presentation of retrocognition by Mrs. Cadel of Johannesburg who is a trained nurse and who writes with a positive sincerity. I shall quote portions from her letter.

"I was living in a small country town. I was sleeping alone in a room and it was a lovely moonlight night. I dropped off to sleep. To this day I cannot say whether what followed was a vision or a dream. I appeared to be looking into the room which I was then occupying, but it was furnished differently. An old iron-and-brass bedstead occupied the middle of the room, an old cane-bottomed chair stood near the bed and an old wash-stand with jug and basin stood near the wall.

"But what seemed to be claiming my attention was a slight man of medium height and of sallow complexion dressed in a policeman's uniform who was standing against the window with one foot up on another old cane-bottomed chair. In his left hand he held a revolver which was levelled at the window. At his side with a terrified look on her face was a slightly-built woman with red hair and brown eyes.

"There was a horrible feeling of tense expectancy. Then I heard the gate opening. It squeaked as it always did when I opened it. There were footsteps and then three knocks at the window. The voice said in Afrikaans : 'Anna open the door. I want to come in.' Three times he knocked and whispered the same urgent request for her to open the door.

"Then the man holding the revolver fired, the woman's shrill scream seemed almost to blast my eardrums. There was the sound of shattered glass—a thud and a groan. The man turned and walked through the other door down the passage, through the kitchen door, down the steps and around the house to where the other man must have been lying.

"I wish I could convey to you the lucidity with which my mind followed his every movement. The steps retreated back up the passage through the other bedroom (where my two children were sleeping) into the room where I was. He looked at the red-haired woman, who was now moaning and crying and said with a sneer, again in Afrikaans : 'Now you bad woman, your lover is dead. You hear, dead' and then he opened the front door leading from the bedroom to the verandah and went out.

"I found myself sitting up in bed, shaking with fright and my heart almost choking me. It was my room again, the moonlight streaming through the window which was intact. "

Mrs. Cadel's investigations revealed that the man and woman had lived there and that a man was found shot for which the wife claimed the responsibility. She said she did it in self-defence. From Mrs. Cadel's letter it appears that this phenomenon never repeated itself while she lived in that house.

This tends to support my theory that retrocognition depends on coincidence of these planes, astral and earth, and to some extent I should think on the thoughts and feelings of the victim.

Perhaps this re-enactment of an earthly scene in astral memory served as a catharsis in the case of the discarnate victim.

Mrs. Cadel went on :

"In 1939 my husband and I attended the celebration of the golden wedding of my parents. Both were in apparent good health and also in good spirits. It was a Friday evening and most of my dream premonitions have occurred on a Friday. During that night I had a dream of my mother. Once again it was a lovely moonlight night. I saw my mother walking along a deserted stretch of beach. The sea was calm and I could see the bottom. I was frantically trying to reach her and was calling out to her to stop. She did stop and turned round to give me a beautiful smile, then said : 'Nae lass, don't try to stop me, I must go my way—'tis time.'

"She then walked away towards the edge of the sea. Again I called and although she turned once to smile at me, she did not speak but walked into the water until it closed over her head. Even then when under the water I could see her walking, so clear was the water. I woke my husband and said : 'Jack my mother is going to die.' He replied : 'Nonsense, we only saw her today and she was all right' and turned over and went to sleep. I did not sleep, but stayed awake awaiting the news which I knew would come and sure enough at about 9 a.m. my father telephoned and said that my mother had suffered a stroke during the night and was unconscious. She never regained consciousness and died ten days later."

The symbolism of this dream is of interest. I have so often heard of dreams from patients which were of a precognitive nature, where they were seeing through water or reading a letter just under the surface of water. Water therefore symbolises another medium of existence, another dimensionality such as the astral. Her mother walked on from the earth and its air into a clear watery medium and kept on walking as if it were the most natural thing in the world to walk under water.

She went on in her letter to tell about her son.

"For years in my dreams when he was a young child, I always had a dream that he was running up the street in front of me in pouring rain; I could never catch up with him, and when I turned the corner he was gone. Since he had nearly died from pneumonia and was subject to severe attacks of croup, I put my dreams down to anxiety neurosis. He grew up a lovely lad, went to the General Botha and later joined the Merchant Navy; at twenty-one he was third mate on a boat.

"At that time my health was very bad and as my son loved me very dearly he relinquished his position and signed on as an A.B.

working his way out to South Africa. A month before he sailed I had a dream which should have warned me. I was standing outside a dilapidated old-fashioned house in a street where all the houses were old and tumble-down with everything grey and horrible. No sign of life and no light.

"I knew that I was waiting for my beloved son, but I did not want him to come to that house and kept saying to myself: 'Don't let him come, oh please don't let him come.' But then I heard his footsteps coming up to me, through the horrible grey light and then his beloved voice, always with a laugh in it, saying 'Well Mom here I am you see. Let's go, shall we?'

"He kissed me and put his hand on the gate to open it. I'd have given anything not to have to open it. We walked with his arm round me up the dusty path to the front door which opened on its own, down the grey passage all mildewed and cobwebby to the kitchen where my mother sat in her armchair in front of the fire, just as she always sat.

"She looked at him smiled and said: 'Well lad it is time you come and look at the clock.' I cried out: 'No Momme, please let him go,' and she replied 'Leave the lad alone it is his time,' and again she looked at the old alarm clock which always stood in our home on the mantel piece above the kitchen stove. It was exactly 8.30 p.m. Well the dream faded. Twenty-one days later on a Tuesday evening my beloved son was killed. Can you imagine what I endured during those twenty-one days?"

On another occasion while working in Port Elizabeth, she was handed a large silver antique-looking brooch to see what impressions she could obtain by means of psychometry. What happened next borders on the fantastic and if one were to accept Mrs. Cadel's statement as true, which I feel reluctant to treat in any other way, then an explanation of her physical reactions is going to be a problem.

She wrote:

"As it was impossible to sit and contemplate the brooch at my desk I went down to the rest-room and sat down on a chintz-covered settee, contemplating the brooch. It was December and hot. I suddenly began to feel icy-cold. The cold sensation was creeping up from my feet and hands and my body began to swell. I developed the most dreadful pain and thought I was dying. Yet I could do nothing."

She must have felt that she had no power to move.

"Evidently the woman who had handed me the brooch became alarmed at my long absence and so came to look for me. She burst into the room and shouted: 'Oh Mrs. C. what's wrong, you look dreadful.' At this I made a supreme effort and flung the brooch from me and gasped : 'You took that brooch from a dead woman who had dropsy and died from heart-failure.'

"She looked at me in amazement and then burst into tears. Between sobs she told me that her mother had had heart-failure and was dropsical and that she had taken the brooch from her mother's dress after her death. It took me two days to get over that experience and the actual swelling of my legs."

I have expressed the opinion that the astral substance, energy system, waveband or whatever term one prefers to facilitate understanding, is a normal constituent of all matter and is also a retainer of memories and impressions. The physical condition of the patient who died of cardiac failure with dropsy, was therefore impressed in nature and feeling on the astral atoms or components of the brooch which she wore.

This must be accepted as a plausible explanation of laws of which our science either in physics or chemistry has no knowledge whatsoever. The hypothesis which I have advanced makes the astral energy system or waveband of vibrations a carrier of memories or images. These in turn when triggered by mind could set up a field of force, a sort of aura in tune with the astral vibrations of the person to whom the object belonged.

All that the mediumistic or psychic person has to do is to concentrate on the object. Mrs. Cadel mentioned "contemplating" it which tends to convey the impression that she gave all her attention to it and was absorbed in its hidden knowledge and conditions.

It is highly probable that the field of force or aura of her own personality potentiated that of the brooch, resonating with it and so entered a frequency rate which tuned in or became identical with the condition of the deceased person prior to her death. In consequence of this identification guided and directed by her mind, her wishes and desires to obtain all the information that she could from the brooch, she placed herself in a receptive or submissive mental state relative to the discarnate owner of the brooch.

She then apparently went into a trance and began to assume the vibrations of pathological energy which were the physical condition of the deceased. The sensations of laboured breathing; the deficiency of air intake and the water retention in the tissues of the legs, as a result of the cardiac insufficiency, all were converted from vibrations into sensations.

The amazing result was that the pathological vibrations could actually become so intense that Mrs. Cadel became almost entranced; that water was retained in her tissues and took two days to become absorbed in a normal manner. I really do not think this would have happened if Mrs. Cadel had not had a strong aura for physical phenomena.

Mr. S., a farmer of Wolseley wrote in Afrikaans about a vision of a tragedy which he could not have perceived by way of his senses. He was driving a small van and his wife and little son sat with him in the cabin while the little servant girl who looked after the baby sat at the back of the van where the "pram" had been fastened to prevent it falling off.

Somewhere along the road his wife asked him why he was driving so very slowly. He told her to wait and not to disturb him as he was absorbed in a vision which showed their little servant girl lying in the road, but in front of the van and not behind it. She was bareheaded and her "kappie" was lying about a hundred yards from her body. She had a smile on her face and he could see this smiling expression most distinctly but blood was coming out of her nostrils; her dress was turned up exposing her thighs and he could see the pattern of her panties; at that moment they came to a gate.

Usually the little servant girl would have jumped off to open the gate. But on this occasion they waited and she did not appear. He then climbed out and found her missing. His wife was terribly upset and they drove back immediately and there in front of the van was the body of the little girl, with all the particulars just as he had seen them in his vision.

Mr. S. has been clairvoyant since his early boyhood years. A vision would suddenly appear and replace the sense impressions of sight of the moment, like a distinct photograph over another indistinct one. The latter would be the image of his normal eyesight and one can conclude the other to be the vision of his astral perception. Many of his visions concerned events which had not materialized.

The number of people with clairvoyant faculties and premonitions or precognitions were decidedly in the majority of those who wrote to me about their experiences. Mrs. van R. of George writing in Afrikaans described an interesting characteristic of her clairvoyant visions which seemed to have been mostly of a precognitive character concerning accidents and deaths. She found that her vision of persons who had died a natural death and who were inwardly at peace about the coming change were white and radiated light. A luminous aura surrounded the form.

On the other hand those who were full of physical life and vigour who met sudden death by unexpected accident were dull-greyish in colour like the haze of a cloud, and inside this dull-grey haze she could discern the features of the physical personality and recognize the individual. The luminosity of natural death of people whose thoughts are of a higher nature is absent in the case of sudden unexpected death. She had often seen visions of people before they committed suicide and these were black.

In these delineations one can attribute the different appearances to the state of individual consciousness. So that the mood and the state of mind and so on are reflected in the aura of the person. It is of interest to observe how often our language unconsciously conveys just these impressions of our minds in certain life situations. The person with hope and courage sees light on his path. The unprepared perplexed and stunned mind finds his outlook clouded and misty and would call it a grey day. The one with suicidal intent and impulse is devoid of hope and courage to face life. To him there is no future, only black despair.

There is however a great compensation in our age for it is amazing to observe how modern psychiatry can snatch the would-be suicide from the very jaws of black despair and within fourteen days sometimes give his brain the enjoyment of the thoughts and moods of light.

The large number of people who have seen with their astral sight those whom they have known during earth life, all have felt convinced that such an experience embodied an element of eternal reality in a moment of understanding, with a realization of inner peace, and firm belief in a continuation of life beyond death. They are religious people and devoted adherents of their churches, but they have found their own interpretations, and most of them have come to the conclusion that they have to exclude from their minds the churchianic idea of people rising from their graves on Judgment Day. Many feel that their experiences have convinced them that this unenlightened conception should be eliminated from churchianic dogma. They all however are loyal to their churches and wish to remain anonymous though differing strongly in their interpretations from these orthodox conceptions.

Experience hence remains the great teacher. For instance Mr. Sch. wrote :

"I could never really believe in life after death. I liked my church and found pleasure in my church activities. But there it ended. The idea of spirit was too intangible for my mind. Then our mother took ill and was in hospital for three months. I visited her regularly before her death. After her funeral that night I slept in the room at home which she had occupied.

I was always a deep sleeper but round about midnight I felt a gentle pressure on my shoulder. It was exercised for a few moments before I fully realized it and woke up wide awake to determine what was the cause of the pressure on my shoulder, when there before my very bed stood my mother. She was clear and distinct in every feature and surrounded by a beautiful luminosity. She smiled so wonderfully happily at me that I was enraptured by the vision and then while still staring at her she was gone and with that vanished my disbelief."

Most of my correspondents wrote in Afrikaans and one could almost gain the impression that the Afrikaans people are extremely psychic. I have often wondered whether it is due to their historical background? One cannot draw definite conclusions but I have found the same thing with the descendants of the 1820 Settlers.

It is as if those people who are bound to the soil of our country sometimes feel deep into the movements of nature. I have before me a letter in Afrikaans which I shall translate as close to the idiom of her linguistic expressions as possible. But since she lives in a small community not far from Port Elizabeth she prefers me not to reveal her address but fortunately there are hundreds of the Strydom clan so that the mere mention of the name will therefore not reveal her identity.

Mrs. Strydom wrote :

"Well doctor I am one of those unfortunate people who came into the world with a faculty that sees the things which are invisible to others. Perhaps it is something natural. I really do not know. My mind cannot grasp the wherefores and whyfores of these purposes of a Higher Hand.

"I must have been very small when I saw a parade of people and ovely things appeared like the sun sometimes suddenly does on a grey and cloudy day. I have a clear memory of a definite vision. I was five years old and woke in the night, and there right in front of my bed sat my granddad. I was so surprised to see 'Oupa' (granddad) there that I called to my mother 'Look Mum here is Oupa.' She lit the lamp but 'Oupa' was gone. Was I surprised! So I said : 'Oupa must have crawled under the bed. He was sitting right here on this chair.' I would not rest and insisted that mother should look under the bed. But we could not find him. Then a few days later 'Oupa' died. Some time later one night while lying awake, I could not sleep and someone came and said farewell to me. I did not know who it was but a few days later I learned that a well-known neighbour had died.

"At the age of fourteen my mother was sick and I had to help her and as I looked towards her bedroom window I saw a light floating, as it were, and it passed the window. This so fascinated me I wondered who it could be, so I peered out and would you believe it, the light came back but the motion was slow; it passed the window quietly and then vanished. My mother died two weeks later.

You can imagine doctor I began to worry about these visions, for always there was some ominous significance. One midday my eldest sister and I stood in the diningroom and as I looked at the front door an old 'Tannie' (Aunt) whom I knew well went past. I told my sister that I had seen the old 'Tannie'. She had gone round to the back of the house. My sister went to look for her and came back to tell me I was crazy there was no one there. Well would you believe it, half-an-hour later a friend came to tell us the 'ou Tannie' had just passed away suddenly. Now tell me doctor how would you explain this?

"There are no queer people in my family. Not one has been insane, then why do people ridicule and jeer at one when you talk about these visions? I can't help this. It is fróm beyond any power of my will. But there is one experience that lives in my mind. That is the one about 'Oom' (Uncle) Moggee. I was feeling terribly restless the whole Sunday. I had a strange intuition that something would happen. I did not know what I was afraid of, but it was not the fear for a person, it was a vague anxiety. I was already seventeen years old but try as I would I could not control this peculiar inner anxiety; this impulse which made it impossible to sit still. I tried to read; I liked reading, but there was my mind running away from the book, seeking something, heaven knew what. At last I became so worked up that I got up and walked about outside in the garden—backwards and forwards—just moving my legs which my feelings would not leave in peace.

"Well while I was in that state of mind Oom Moggee came past the garden. He knew all about my visions and premonitions and used to tease me about them. But when he saw me in the garden he stopped and said : 'Pop, are you afraid of a vision again? Why do you roam about so restlessly in the garden?' I answered : 'Yes, I am afraid.' Well would you believe me doctor that same night I woke—I was wide awake—and there before me stood Oom Moggee. Those eyes were so wide open, staring at me and there was his body, and it had a streaming faint glow around it. I knew then that Oom Moggee would die soon.

"Somehow, being young I fell asleep but woke early and dressed as quickly as I could and ran to the house of an 'ou Tannie' nearby. We understood each other, but as I ran into her house she first scolded me for running in the rain without an overcoat. I did not reply to her scolding but burst out in excitement and said 'Tannie, Oom Moggee is going to die. I saw him life-like last night but he was in a spirit body."

"The Tannie was so taken aback that she said : 'Our heavenly Father my child, you must not say such a thing. Did you not know that Oom Moggee had a haemorrhage from his lung late last night and the doctor was called?' I told her that I knew nothing about any illness of Oom Moggee's. I only saw him in my room in a beautiful body. Well doctor, Oom Moggee died three weeks later.

"There is something else that I want to tell you, and you may laugh if you like, but I believe that places acquire something from people. There is something which hangs about a person like an invisible part of himself which I can feel. I can sense this in their homes, and I know when people are sincere. This atmosphere which surrounds them tells me these things.

"Tell me doctor, what sort of person am I? I have been most unhappy when in my impulsive youth I blurted out these thoughts about my visions, now I am older and wiser and look out before I lay myself open to common ridicule. I did not make myself. God made me like this. How can I help it when I naturally see those who have died come back and smilingly visit the places which they loved.

"But I will tell you what has always come to my mind. It has always appeared to me when I see these phantoms of the dead, that there is something mental, some thought, or desire maybe, some message which keeps on making them seek their old habitations because they want to convey these thoughts to people living. That is why I say, they do not seem to understand the new life these people who wander around. It should really be far more interesting over there than here where we have so many troubles. Or don't you agree doctor? I have really written far too much, but let me tell you. I don't know you and yet I enjoyed writing all these things for it seemed that unseen friends were prompting me. Goodbye and good luck."

I have curtailed this letter which flowed so smoothly and amusingly in Afrikaans, and yet so deeply impregnated with sincere and almost reverent thought that one cannot doubt its authenticity. In most of these clairvoyant visions the significance was always some death in the family or circle of friends. The Afrikaans letters on this particular subject all have this ominous meaning with the happening coming later as confirmation.

The traditional Afrikaans pattern of life has always been to help each other, to nurse their sick fellowmen on farms, and to sit up nights on end to serve each other with deep sympathy. They lived into each other's lives, sharing their emotions of suffering, as a corporate body whose feelings were communal. There has been since yonder time a mutual struggle for self-preservation and I have often during my years in medical practice admired this tremendous self-sacrificing spirit among the rural Afrikaners. Perhaps it is due to the cultivation of this attitude of mind and empathy, that self-preservation plays such a prominent part in the precognitive clairvoyant visions or my Afrikaans correspondents. One cannot however fail to observe from their letters their profound reverence for life.

Mrs. Alex. writing from Pretoria in Afrikaans described how deeply attached she was to her mother. This feeling did not make her dependent and she managed her own house and family. But there was a bond between her mother and herself which always gave her such happiness and contentment when they were together and she had often thought that should her mother die she would feel this void very much. She never gave life hereafter any thought. Then she heard rappings in a corner of her house which could not be explained and thereafter she saw lights which always mysteriously disappeared and for which no one could give a reason. Then came the news of her mother's sudden heart attack. This affected her in such a manner that before she could undertake the trip to her mother she retched and retched for hours. She arrived at the sickbed to find her mother very exhausted. She opened her eyes and slowly reached out for her daughter's hand and said: "You must not sorrow over me. There is no need for grief, I am deeply happy inside. Try and listen with me, I am hearing the most beautiful music. It seems to be drawing me, but it is far far away," and then she breathed her last.

Now in spite of her mother's last words, Mrs. Alex. could not stop grieving for her. She could not reconcile herself to her loss, and she could not find solace in the idea of her mother's happiness in some non-physical state. She wept almost daily when her thoughts turned to her mother. Then one evening, feeling very sad upon going to bed, she ultimately fell asleep, and had a most striking and clear dream. She found herself on top of a high mountain and down below in the most beautiful deep green valley she had ever seen, were little white goats. But they were unlike any goat she had ever seen in her life. She remembered making this comparison in her dream. They fascinated her because they were so milk-white, so smooth and so beautifully formed moving with such grace and rhythm that she climbed down the mountainside to get closer to them.

But as she reached the foot of the mountain, a beautiful diamond-like sparkling stream ran almost at her feet. The running water and its scintillating reflections and bouncing little drops or globules all seemed to be animated by a strange sort of life. She was spellbound in her dream for the water and the goats and the landscape all seemed alive with spirit. At least this she felt.

Then she looked up and there at the side of the diamond-sparkled flowing water stood her mother, completely radiant.

She ran to her full of joy and flung her arms round her mother's neck and hugged and hugged her with intense happiness; almost a state of ecstasy.

After a moment her mother said to her : "Do you not remember your promise not to grieve for me? I do not want your heart to be heavy with sorrow for me. I am very happy and peacefully contented here. Now go back to your life—you will remember this experience in all its gracefulness." With this the dream faded and she woke free from all grief and sorrow. She only regretted that she did not have the ability to put into words the exquisite experience of the dream. "Did I really meet my mother in the next world?"

I too have wondered whether Mrs. Alex.'s dream could have been an astral flight to some other region of life on the astral. A large number of people described dreams which, because of their coherent vividness and normal flow of events, they considered could have been psychic experiences other than dreams. Premonitions were often deduced from such dreams.

A Mr. du Plessis writing in Afrikaans described how his little girl of ten came into their bedroom one morning and said : "Daddy last night I was awake in my sleep. My body was dead but I walked about the house. I was on the stoep and actually came to look at you sleeping and then went back to my body." He ended his letter by saying that "the apple does not fall far from the tree," as he is a most vivid dreamer and meets all sorts of people who are dead in his dreams and they discuss many interesting subjects. There were times when he went on long journeys in his dreams and travelled on trains and ships but there was never anything illogical and irrational about his dreams.

Mr. du Plessis did not know that his little daughter's description of her experience was in all probability a typical astral projection. Maybe his dream journeys are forms of astral consciousness and experience. I shall refer to some South African experiences of this nature later on.

Mr. L. writing from Durban described her psychic experiences as follows :

"I have had many psychic experiences and believe in a guardian spirit who has never let me down. My clairvoyant visions have been most unexpected and occurred even in crowded places at times. My mother who had had an unhappy married life had died when I was very young. About a year after her death I was in a crowded street in broad daylight when she suddenly appeared to me looking radiantly happy.

I was at that time living with my brother and his wife and I had an uncle of about fifty. Then one night I had a life-like imagery that the house was upset by my uncle's death. I told his wife who laughed and said that he was very well. Then later the same day my brother 'phoned me to say that my uncle had dropped dead at table. From that time I had clear premonitions of accidents, deaths and other disasters concerning our family or friends. Besides, I must mention that during my nursing days, I often could feel a strange power flowing through me to my patients.

The appearance of a phantom of the dead is well protrayed in this letter from Mrs. R. She wrote in Afrikaans :

"My husband, a constable in the South African Police went out one evening to look out for people who were shooting game by means of spotlights. I was alone at home with my two small children. I was very nervous and afraid of being left alone so it was well after midnight before I fell into a slumber. Suddenly I woke and as I opened my eyes I saw a man in his working clothes next to my bed. I was speechless with fear and the cold sweat poured from me. The person was my brother-in-law. I tried to speak to ask what he wanted for in spite of the darkness I could see him distinctly and recognize his features. Then in a very tired, I should say exhausted voice he said : 'Clara please give Koos (his little boy) a piece of bread' and at once he vanished. I felt that I was going to develop a heart attack I was so upset and my heart was pounding so much that I trembled all over.

While still in this emotional upheaval I heard a knock at the front door. Naturally I thought that my husband had returned from his patrol and without taking the torch or matches, I just ran to the door to meet him. But it was not my husband, it was a friend who came to tell us that my brother-in-law had died suddenly from a heart attack."

In studying this correspondence from people in all walks of life I noticed significantly how the feelings of people or their mood-states, to be more precise, were affected beforehand by these psychic phenomena. The premonitory type which heralds bad news was not infrequently ushered in by a phase of depression and anxiety. It seems as if this inner awareness of a precognitive nature is happening on a subconscious level of the mind. This could be the case if the astral personality is the true primary Perceiver of these events, as I believe it is, except where it is capable of perceiving an astral separation or projection of the deceased as in the case of Mrs. R. This lady saw her brother-in-law, who in symbolic language really asked her to keep a motherly eye on Koos when he employed the phrase "give him a piece of bread."

Where these clear visions or phantoms do not immediately express their intention, I found in a large number of letters, a fairly prolonged prodromal state of mind of an unhappy or a restless nature. Mrs. Paige for instance writes as follows :— "I get very depressed and feel like crying all the time. This happened every time a member of my family passed away, even some time before they take ill or meet with an accident." One can assume that this is a feeling-state of the astral personality which is aware of the emotional reaction which the external mind would experience. It then transmits this feeling to the outer mood-state before the act of knowing occurs.

The next case is of a different nature, but indicates that some compelling force directed Mr. Thompson. He wrote that four years ago he was informed that one of the military personnel on Robben Island has been drowned. They found no trace of his body. Mr. Thompson being in the Transvaal felt a strange urge, an attraction in fact to go and find the remains of this man drowned off Robben Island.

During September of that year he was on holiday at the Cape and so he spent a weekend on Robben Island. Wherever he asked he met the reply that no remains of the drowned man had been found. He then proceeded to the beach and stood at the cross which had been erected in the man's memory. After a while he felt a tremendous pull or urge to go to a crevice between the rocks, and there he found the bones of the right leg of the drowned man.

He took the bones to the lighthouse and the Officer Commanding the Garrison was summoned. By that time Mr. Thompson knew that somewhere along the beach were the rest of the man's body. The next day the search revealed these remains in unlooked-for places.

Now the drowned man was apparently no friend of Mr. Thompson's and yet he became obsessed with the idea away up in the Transvaal that he should find the body, and the subsequent events showed a peculiar form of inner-thought-directive that led him to discover the remains. What would be the reasons for excluding any influence from the discarnate self of the victim?

Candidly, if one has to account for this peculiar motivation of a stranger's actions which became so urgent that he had to respond to them, then one must accept influences which did not come from those living on earth at the time. One can assume that the victim of the drowning was greatly affected by the idea that he had not had a proper burial. Who knows but that his creedal conception of life and death made a burial of his remains a condition of his happiness on the next plane!

CHAPTER VI

VISIONS AND PREMONITIONS

Mrs. K. wrote to me:— "I feel I must relate an amazing experience which I once had. We were farming near Wellington, and I had some chickens in an outbuilding on the farm. One very hot noonday I was tapping water into a watering can to take to my chickens. I was expecting my first child and was seven months pregnant. As I was about to move away carrying the can, I saw a robed golden presence standing next to me and he said :— "Don't take the water to the chickens, call the servant."

I thought to myself :— "Am I getting a little crazy because of my pregnancy?" Anyway I went through the gate and the golden presence walked beside me telling me not to go, but to send the servant. I ignored him and continued towards the outbuildings. He suddenly stepped in front of me and would not allow me to pass. Putting the watering can down I went back to the house and asked the servant to take the water to the chickens. I sat on a low wall and watched her take the can; I was deeply puzzled.

A few moments later she dashed out of the building, her skirts lifted up and her cap jerked from her head, and waving it in her hand she came screaming terrified and shuddering towards me. "What is the matter?" I shouted as out of breath and trembling she explained that a huge Cape cobra had been sleeping under the water receptacle and as she moved it, the snake flung itself up in a fright and struck at her but just missed her feet. She almost leapt into the air in order to escape from the building.

One can imagine what effect such a fright would have had on Mrs. K. in her condition. This experience would be interpreted by a large number of people as the warning of a guardian spirit. Many of my correspondents felt as though on occasions of danger there was an extraneous influence, some presence but not perceptible, who sounded a warning note telepathically setting up feelings of anxiety and caution.

Mrs. K. records another experience which I am sure many will class among the fairy tales of life. Still one cannot dismiss this story because of the honesty and sincerity of her letter; besides she would hardly, with her name and address known to me have sent me a fabrication.

She went on to say :— "My little daughter was born with a cough, and as time progressed this developed into bronchitis and asthma. We had her tonsils removed by a specialist and we used every remedy which was prescribed and even sent her away to the Transvaal for a whole year. She was under doctors for eight years in Wellington as well.

At last we bought a cottage at Bain's Kloof, the original old Toll House, and I went to live up there in the mountain air with two of my younger children. My husband and my eldest son of ten years were left on the farm with a coloured woman to care for them. We had been up at Bain's Kloof for two months but the child remained bedridden and seriously ill. The local doctor told me he had not had such a case before; there was not a patch of her lungs which was not congested and affected.

Then came June the 2nd—dawn was breaking and it was her birthday. I was lying in the bed beside her. For most of the night I had listened in despair to her struggle for breath. She was exhausted but still had the will to live. Then I was overcome and felt so utterly helpless. It was her eighth birthday and never had she had one without suffering.

I suddenly called to God and said :— "Oh God it is her birthday, eight years of bitter suffering. We have tried everything. God you know what will cure her, tell me, tell me what to do." As this cry of anguish left my lips there in the dark room before my eyes appeared words, illuminated words, mentioning a preparation of garlic extract. I leapt out of bed, dressed hurriedly and found myself running all the way to the nearest telephone. I told my husband to get me a bottle of this preparation at all cost.

That night we started the child on it. After four days the lungs were less congested and within fourteen days her shoulders had lost their asthmatic bearing and a little later her lungs were clear and we returned to the farm. She became so well that she was able to attend school. She is now a fine strong normal girl. She took the medicine for two years and still does whenever she has a cold. When she pulls a face I remind her of the doctor who prescribed it and then she drinks it with gratitude."

Now it is not my intention to advertise any remedy so I have left out the specific name. I happen to know that this remedy was extensively taken by sufferers of chest complaints, especially croup, bronchitis and asthma. Many people swore by it and others found no benefit. Today it is not as popular as it used to be according to well-informed chemists.

We must assume that Mrs. K.'s story is authentic and the truth. The dramatic change in the child, living in the same environment, after taking the extract of garlic could simply be considered a case of an effective cure. But it raises deeper issues and questions. Was the vibration of healing as an inherent property of garlic not augmented and greatly surcharged by a frequency rate of energy generated by the psychic mother? How much of this field of force radiated by her, coupled with its inflow from cosmic sources was absorbed by the extract of garlic?

One cannot answer such a question in an objective manner, but when one is reminded of my experience with the little primula of flowers which healed my daughter's throat, then it becomes easier to accept and understand the existence of mysterious wavebands of energy, which could be magnetised by the power of thought. When one's thoughts move in a poetical frame then a cosmic consciousness seems to loom up as the source of these strange happenings.

Anyway I think that these miraculous instances which occur for some people, but with the same remedy failing with others, strongly support my hypothesis that there are human conductors of certain healing vibrations, and that these vibrations are inherent in our beings in varying potentialities, but can at times be augmented by supernormal psychic means. How many of our daily physical remedies are not enhanced in value by the same means as employed by Mrs. K.?

Returning to premonitions, Mrs. W. of Rosebank, Johannesburg, wrote :— "While in Lourenco Marques on business on February 22nd, I had a most realistic dream, albeit shocking. I was in a clean all-white room, with a very high ceiling and everything was smooth and rounded. I saw part of a large bath, with a drying rack suspended over it containing white laundry. One piece of this washing was an old white blouse of mine and blood was seeping on to it fresh and red. I looked up and saw that the blood was pulsating out of a corner of the ceiling. I woke trying desperately to get into the ceiling. I was perturbed about this dream as we had to fly home Friday the 24th but did not mention it to my chief."

Her trip was uneventful however and she described her dream to a friend. But on Sunday, February 26th at 6.30 p.m. she received a frantic call. "My son aged nineteen years and a friend had been climbing on the rock face at Hartebeestpoort dam hoping to save time in getting to the "Cosmos" side to look at a boat for sale. The rock gave way and he crashed twenty-five to thirty feet into the spillway basin on concrete rocks. His injuries were terrible. I saw him at about 8.15 p.m.—the blood was still pulsating through the padded bandage on his knee." Her son recovered except for a stiff ankle.

This dream took place four days before her son's accident and the chief characteristics were the oozing blood, fresh and red to convey the accident idea and then the white rounded room and the white laundry signifying hospital. Four days before it happened these impressions appeared in a dream. Where did they come from and who was the knower of their significance? Several mothers who had been closely attached to members of their families have written of dreaming about their children's misfortunes and even misdemeanours, always before these took place.

Mrs. Ada Donnelly of Johannesburg described her premonition of her mother's death which included a vision of words. One evening while going from Johannesburg to Klerksdorp she and her husband decided to stop at her mother's place in Potchefstroom because, being Mothers' Day, she had bought her a special cake. When she entered her mother's room the old lady was in bed reading her Bible; she was dressed all in white, also the bedclothes appeared spotlessly white, and while looking at her mother she saw written across her face the words :— "The peace that passeth all understanding." At this she drew back. Naturally the experience was disturbing, uncanny and unexpected.

Her mother however noticed her reaction and said :— "Come in Ada, what is the matter?" That evening on the way home she told her husband what she had seen and added that she knew her mother would not spend Christmas with them as arranged, but would pass away. Her husband however considered her suspicions unfounded. But in spite of his dismissal of her fears she felt so convinced that she made arrangements for her sister's child to stay with her granny. Then came the day they were to fetch her mother for her Christmas holiday but that forenoon a telegram came— "Mother passed away this morning."

Mrs. Donnelly also described brighter precognitive experiences. "Now you may remember that July 1954 when *Cesi Bon* won the Durban July? Well the Monday night before the race I woke my husband at about 2 a.m. and said to him :— "Remember this, I have just been to the Durban July Race. Somebody handed me a piece of paper and on it in a childish handwriting in carbon was written "*Cesi Bon* won the Durban July," and then somebody shouted "Yes Radlington second and Spey Bridge third," and then another voice shouted "No Spey Bridge second and Radlington third." After the race was run I heard the same mistake made by Ernie Duffield over the air and if I remember correctly it was a photo-finish. Now this was not like a dream. I was just there alive; it was vivid and real. Naturally we cashed in and I told all my friends. Well they just did not believe me but were very sorry afterwards."

One observes that the written means of communication and presentation occurred twice in Mrs. Donnelly's experience; once across her mother's face and then the piece of paper at the Durban July. The latter event was perceived in such detail just as it occurred, especially the part of the radio announcer. The rational conclusion is that the whole event was already in existence, winner and all, at least five days before the time. This aspect of precognition always raises one of the most profound problems for understanding our wills and our existence in this world.

I now wish to relate one of many personal precognitive perceptions. It is my custom to walk at least four miles early every morning, before preparing for my professional day. One morning while reading the morning paper, I noticed that a Herald snake had been acquired by the Port Elizabeth Snake Park. I must add that I have no special interest in snakes, except to give them a wide berth. But while just glancing at the words "Herald Snake", I suddenly saw in my mind a large vicious puffadder rearing itself right in front of my feet. I immediately became aware that this was a premonition, and that I would encounter a puffadder on my walk.

Accordingly I decided that I would not go anywhere near bushes and would avoid the Baakens River Reserve. I would walk on the golf course along the fairways. At least, I thought, this would be the most unlikely place for puffadders. I duly walked briskly inhaling the pure clean air, far removed from the exhaust and diesel engine pollution of the city streets.

I was walking along deep in thought, for these were always my moments when my thinking was unfettered by extraneous disturbances. Suddenly I heard a hiss, and as I leapt back there next to the green in a little footpath was the half-raised body and the broad vicious head of a huge puffadder. Another few inches and I would have trodden on it so "the best laid schemes o mice and men gang aft agley." The puffadder of course could have been lying there sunning itself when I got the impression in my bedroom but its reaction to my presence had not yet occurred. The question is did I see all that happened on another dimensionality? The event was there, I had only to come across it.

There are persons who predominantly have astral vision or clairvoyant impressions of something portentous. Mrs. D. Jones of Sasolburg is one of these psychic sensitives. I have often wondered whether there is not a subconscious anxiety determining extrasensory perceptions of this nature. Writing in Afrikaans she described such a peculiar experience.

"On one occasion a friend and I were sitting on the stoep and in one corner was an empty chair. Looking at this corner I saw to my amazement a skeleton sitting on this chair with his legs crossed. I did not say anything but made some excuse to get away and so suggested that we should go and lie down in her bedroom. We did this and each took a book to read.

"But as I placed my hand under my head to support it whilst

reading, someone repeatedly pulled it away. In the end I just could not stand it any more and so got off the bed and told my friend of my experiences. I thought it was a premonition of a death, and sure enough three days later she received a telegram informing her that her grandmother had died.

"On another occasion I was living with a widowed lady. Then one day, apropos of nothing, I looked up into the corner of the room and there I saw a beautiful face of a lovely little girl, but her eyes were closed as if in sleep. One morning two weeks later we heard a queer noise of clinking glasses in the sittingroom, but when we investigated we found nothing had been disturbed. A few moments later word came that the lady's lovely little granddaughter had died."

She went on to say :

"The visions which I see are symbolic and they vary from time to time. On occasions I have seen balls of light extremely bright, and then again I would sit in a room and it would become misty and greyish, while at other times I would see the back of some person for a moment. I have heard groaning as well, so that I do not only see things. On one occasion the groaning was followed within two days by the death of my beloved grandfather as well as that of my uncle.

"Once while boarding with some people in Vereeniging I went home for a weekend to my parents on the farm and while there on the Saturday afternoon I saw a picture like a cinematograph of a truck being driven by someone and I saw a child fall off it, followed by a mattress as if they were flying through the air. The next day when I arrived at Vereeniging my landlady informed me that they had gone camping and a child and a mattress had fallen off the truck exactly as I had seen it happen."

The dramas which are lived in the minds of people subject to ominous precognition are seldom appreciated by those of us who merely learn of such experiences "second hand" as it were. The following Afrikaans letter from a lady who calls herself "Mamoesa" is of profound interest in showing the anxiety reactions and restless depression which often accompany the precognitive awareness of some impending distress or tragedy.

Because of one particular experience in this letter the correspondent wishes to remain anonymous.

"I have since my earliest years had an uncanny sense of knowing things before they happen. Always there was the impression of some greater self within me knowing or sensing the event, and then a part of my mind became afraid of the consequence, before my brain knew what it really was.

"Three years ago my husband died suddenly without any

complaint. Outwardly and in his actions he appeared healthy and strong. But weeks before his death a strange restless fear gripped me. At night I who usually slept very well, would lie awake as if awaiting the approach of something soul-disturbing. At last I could not keep it to myself any longer and I said to him 'My man there is something terrible going to happen, but I don't know what.' He teased me and said I was probably being haunted and laughed it away.

"At that time my one daughter was on holiday in Durban. I felt that I wanted her home and I pleaded with my husband to allow me to send her a telegram to come home immediately. But he considered it unreasonable to spoil her hard-earned holiday for reasons of my imagination and was adamant that I should not disturb her with my fears. But my anxiety increased and became worse, until it became so irresistible that I had to send the telegram. I did so without my husband's knowledge. The next morning she arrived at Pretoria about 9 o'clock and while she was in the taxi coming home I received the message that my husband had died suddenly at work.

"Some years later one of my sons aged ten years went to Durban without my knowledge. That night I discovered that my child was missing and we could not find him anywhere. None of us had any idea that he had secretly gone with some people. After three days I was really terribly distressed and was dozing off to sleep when I dreamed. All right I shall call it a dream, but it was an appearance and a conversation. My husband came to me and said : 'Old girl what is our little boy doing in Durban in a tea-room bioscope?'

"I immediately called my children and told them what their father had said. My son, daughter and I left that same night and drove straight through to Durban. We arrived there at six in the morning. My son who was driving felt quite exhausted and went to sleep while my daughter and I rushed to this tea-room bioscope described by my husband. It was just interval when we went in and there were about a hundred people in the place. The light was on and there sat my little boy. Who sent me there? Was it not my husband from the other side, even if he appeared in a dream?

"Some years before that we lived at a certain place in an old house. My husband worked on the railways. The second night that we slept in that house after our transfer I jumped out of bed with my heart beating in my throat. I could swear that I saw and felt a little baby boy sitting on my feet. In spite of protests from my husband, and we were very happy pals, I refused to sleep without the light burning during that night. The next morning I dismissed it as a nightmare and even laughed at myself and forgot the whole thing.

"But that night round about midnight I again got the fright of my life. There was the child once more sitting on my feet. I gave such a scream of terror that my husband nearly fell out of the bed, and our children were all awakened and came running to see what had happened. Again I kept the light burning until the morning. By this time I was confoundedly fed-up with these nightmares and hallucinations as my husband called them. That night at about the same time, the exact picture repeated itself. But this time I saw the child, a little boy, very plainly. I even saw how the tears shone in his little eyes but unfortunately I always screamed so impulsively before I could observe things more closely. After the fifth appearance of this child at night, always sitting on my feet, I refused to spend another minute in that house.

"I maintained that the child was haunting the house and strangely believed that it was buried somewhere near as a result of some tragedy. I told everybody because I felt that I wanted to find his burial-place. But look as I would and where I could there was not a grave for miles around the place. I could not give up the idea of finding this child's burial-place, and at last confided my tremendous urge to my neighbour because others ridiculed my nightly experience. She however was a sensible and understanding person and said she also felt that there was a reason behind this child's appearance. She would help me.

"The two of us searched all over the yard of the house but found nothing. Then something directed me to the house itself and I examined the floor-boards. My husband and male friend stood there and laughed and laughed because I was so obsessed I was even loosening the old floor-boards. It was a very old railway cottage and there was a deep space beneath the floor-boards and the earth. My friend and I ignored the menfolk. We lifted up the planks and climbed down into the space beneath. We were brave, it was of course broad daylight, and the men were with us even if they were making fun of us. I raked around in the loose earth when I hooked an old perished or rotten blanket.

"At once they were all interested and the men came to see. I went on raking and then found a child's skull and some small bones. I took the bones in my hands. They were the little bones of a baby and I even found the mouldy little shirt round the little chest bones. Immediately I knew what had happened. I wanted to report the discovery but my husband would not hear of it. We buried the bones again where we had found them and nailed the planks in position but that same evening we were out of that house with all that we possessed. We went to live miles away from that house. Yet for nights this same little baby boy came to me and always I woke with a scream."

One wonders whether this baby's astral presence would have been perceived if "Mamoesa" had not been a psychic sensitive. It was indeed a gruesome find, but the reappearance of the child long afterwards at different places rather suggests that "Mamoesa" had a power for attracting the discarnate body who seemed to have been actuated by a need to find a mother-being.

Was he a little orphan left in the charge of someone who did not care or was he illegitimate and met his end through neglect and under-nourishment? The dynamic need to be loved and to find the protection of some mother-being had probably bound him to the denser regions of the astral, from which "Mamoesa" might have been able to free him if love and not fear had dominated her feelings. Most of us go about our daily tasks quite unconscious of these psychological calamities and tragedies linking the feelings of man with unknown regions.

From Ceres district I received a letter from a Mrs. A. and I give here a translation from the Afrikaans.

"A friend of mine was seriously ill. I had a bit of a conflict and for personal reasons did not want to visit him during those days of his illness. But while he was still alive and in his bed at home I saw him walking in at my front door. I knew he was extremely ill with cancer of the lungs so that he could not possibly come to me. Yet there he was as if completely his physical self. He walked to my room and went to lie down on my bed. I stood in front of the bed and placed my hand on his forehead asking him whether he had much pain and if there was anything which I could do for him. He did not answer and just vanished.

On another occasion I saw him sitting in my kitchen and then he got up and walked backwards and forwards, to and fro, as if he were in great pain. Then one Saturday evening I again saw him life-like but somehow he appeared very perplexed or worried. He died the next day. After his death I saw him once more and thereafter he never appeared again."

The phantom during life could have been a thoughtform or an automatic astral projection because Mrs. A. did not visit him. She had her reasons, but the attraction between the two persons and her sensitive psychic state evidently facilitated his appearance from time to time within the range of her field of force. She understood these phantom phenomena as forebodings of his death.

Premonitions in children are always of interest because of the innocent nature of this type of thought. Mr. Herman Snyman reported in *Die Vaderland se Sondagblad* the foreboding vision of a four-year old. "Little Deon Els came running out of breath into his mother's room, very excited with wide staring eyes. Mammy, the four-year old boy called out. I have just seen Daddy. He was with me in the room and he said that he was coming to fetch me before the end of the year." Fifteen hours later Deon was involved in a motor-car accident and died under narcosis in hospital. His father had died a few months before Deon."

Here then we have the simple understanding of a child who at four was most excited at the idea of leaving this world to join his Daddy. The events that followed and the manner in which he related his experience to his mother leaves little room for doubt that his father's appearance was to prepare him for the fact that he would be met by him on the other side.

There are people whose premonitions take the form of visions, and others again just experience intense fear and unhappiness, whereas others plainly hear voices forbidding them to do something or other. At one time I thought this could be one's deeper self with a wider consciousness operating on another dimensionality forewarning one. But a number of letters detailing the experiences of people, especially those who saw warning phantoms have shown that these apparitions have been recognised as members of the family or friends who were deceased.

This type of evidence leaves one with the conclusion that one's self-preservation is a psychic force which perhaps telepathically becomes the concern of those discarnate beings still linked by bonds of friendship and affection. Or have we each some guardian being in the unseen domain who at times tries to influence us against unpleasant or disastrous actions?

Mr. J. A. Nardin of Port Elizabeth wrote me a charming letter which showed that even as a child he had his astral sight and hearing well developed. It almost compared with his physical sight and hearing. But his parents dismissed these impressions of his as nightmares or just vivid dreams. Then years later while working in Johannesburg, in fact it was in 1936, he developed a toothache on his way to work. As he was waiting for his tram a voice distinctly and clearly said to him : Don't go to work today. You have a toothache." But he decided toothache or not he should attend to his job.

The voice however became more insistent and he almost felt like turning back. At last he reached the employees' entrance of the Carlton Hotel, and then the voice said very loudly : "Don't go to work today." He entered the building and never heard that voice again. The same evening he had his right hand mangled in a mincing machine and it was so serious that it had to be amputated the following day. He thought that in mental association with him was a discarnate being conscious of the accident to come who tried to prevent it by warning him.

Most of the letters which I received contained the request for anonymity for some reason or other, but they were all so tangibly honest and sincere that one cannot fail to accept them as real experiences. Mrs. N. wrote in Afrikaans :

"I was tremendously worried and had a terrific problem. I could not sleep as I could not see any immediate solution, and the only course open to me was not one that I felt I could take. I did not know where to turn. So in the dead of the night, sleepless and very upset with worries I was lying staring into the darkness hoping for what I knew not, when suddenly I heard my name called.

"Yes, it was called by the voice of my late father who died several years before. It was his voice—the tone of the voice and the manner of pronouncing my name was his. We had loved each other dearly. As I lay there flabbergasted by this voice which I had heard, I saw a cloud form in my room and there within this cloud stood the clear outline of my father; his bald head and every feature and characteristic as I knew him in life. I was stunned with amazement.

"The cloudy outline of his figure was bluish-white and seemed alive or moving like moving rays circulating around him. Again he called my name and said : 'Do you find this life too much for yourself, and do you want me to fetch you away?' I said : 'No father I shall try and solve my problems,' and with that he vanished. The solution which I found the next day had several aspects I had never thought of."

She went on to describe that her son had a very clever and pretty little daughter of seven. They all adored this little girl. On a particular day, Mrs. N. bought herself a pot of face cream and placed it on her dressing table. That evening she and her husband were sitting on the bed talking when the screwed-on lid of the pot of face cream just jumped off and ran around the room bouncing over things. Her husband laughed and said jokingly that she was so keen about beautifying herself that she had acquired a ghost.

She screwed on the lid as tightly as possible but no sooner had she placed the pot of cream on the table when to their utter astonishment the lid jumped off the pot, rolled on the floor and circled round and round, bouncing in the manner that a cart wheel in flight would do. She immediately felt that something would happen, some tragedy for she was aware that the behaviour of the lid was a foreboding. Two days later her adorable little granddaughter was killed in an accident.

A lady wrote that during the last war she had a son at the front. One morning she walked into her room and saw a misty cloud-like column in the corner, then the form and face of her son appeared looking very sad and miserable. After the war she learned that on that day four of his companions had been shot as spies but his execution was postponed for a few days for the purpose of questioning. Just before he was te be executed the Americans arrived and released him. He recalled that while awaiting his turn to be shot he had thought intently of her. Here then was a projection of a thoughtform which was seen as a phantom of her son.

Mrs. Mey wrote from Benoni :

"I have always had advanced knowledge of death of members of my family or friends through dreams. For example I was living in England for a few years and saw clearly a friend of mine who resided in George, Cape Province fully dressed in evening clothes drop dead. My mother who lived in Oudtshoorn at the time confirmed this by letter.

"My husband and I returned to South Africa and lived at Koegasbrug in the Northern Cape. In September 1951 I had the most vivid dream of my father-in-law standing at the foot-end of the bed, trying to speak to me. The noise he made was terrible and I could not understand him, except for the word "will". His face turned purplish blue and he dropped to the floor. I awoke terrified and woke my husband. We learned later that he had died of a stroke on the night of my dream. What is more the family could find no will but we knew there was one. We knew that one had been made.

"While living at Koegasbrug the dreams became more frequent, not only of death notices but also of premonitions of accidents. In the end my friends would not come near me if I talked of dreams. They told me to shut up. They were frightened because my dreams always came true.

"For instance I dreamed of our neighbour's little girl and in the dream were visions of an operating theatre, screaming ambulance sirens and people running about. After each of these dreams I would wake terrified. I called on my neighbour Mrs. V.D.B. and told her to keep the little girl in the yard as I had had one of my queer dreams. By 1 p.m. the ambulance went screaming down the mine's one main road. I was working in the mine office and was summoned to find the District Surgeon. He was almost fifty miles away. The rush and confusion was exactly as in my dream. The little girl had eaten some pips from a seed-box containing Belladonna poison. She hovered between life and death but fortunately survived. After this I was regarded almost as a witch.

"Then a very close friend of my husband's was involved in an accident. He was taken to Cape Town but we knew he would not recover. Then came the night of his death and he appeared in my dream, real and life-size. He told me that he would be passing over that night and asked us to help his wife in her need. The next morning we learned of his death.

"Some time later we moved to Benoni and one evening when I slept at my sister's place it happened again. My mother appeared at the foot of my bed. She called to me and told me not to be frightened. She had been sick in hospital in Oudtshoorn but had recovered and was due to leave for home. But she told me that she was very sorry that she won't see her home with her physical self again as she was going to die at 10 a.m. on the next day and that we must please take care of my kid brother aged fourteen years. Before I could speak she had vanished. Again as usual I was wide awake and frightened to death and shivering.

"I woke my husband and told him and he asked me not to say anything to my sister. The whole day I contained myself but that evening I could not keep it to myself any longer. I told her of my dream but she dismissed it saying that by that time Mammy would be safely home from the hospital. We arrived at her house to find the servant holding a telegram. Mother had died that morning at 10 o'clock as she had told me in my dream."

It is of interest to note that the diviners or isanuses among the Amaxosa people, also the witchdoctors or amagqira place great reliance on their dream communications. They believe that the ancestral spirits communicate by means of the dream mind. In their dreams they usually describe visions of their ancestral spirits. These communications could of course be telepathic contact with discarnate members of the tribe. Some of the visions were described as objective and clear portraying features and characteristics known during physical life. One wonders whether these Amaxosa dream communications with the dead are not perhaps a form of contact on the astral plane.

These dreams and forms of psychic communication show that the events of tomorrow are intimately linked with one's instinctive concern for self-preservation. The evidence suggests that those who are intimately emotionally associated with one's life somehow find channels of communications which bypass the sensory faculties.

The isanuse may go to sleep with his problem, or the desire for knowledge of something required by someone. Then in his dreams he receives a communication from one he acknowledges as an ancestral spirit. I think this has the same significance as what is known as a guardian spirit. Hence he is shown events which will come about in time. These are always seen in the dream in the same manner as they eventually take place.

Often one observes the morbid trend of some of these premonitions be they in dreams or visions seen clairvoyantly. And one is somewhat inclined to accept that the predominant precognitive trends concern tragedies, deaths and mournful scenes. But I have received a large number of letters in which the precognitive or premonitory impressions also concern the more pleasant tones of life, such as success in business, in social life and in the fulfilment of ambition.

One has to conclude from this evidence that the warning aspect of precognitive experience is perhaps more frequent because of the mood or state of mind of the recipient. In other words that all our problems are wrapped in anxiety and therefore these dramatic subjective experiences are more often remembered and talked about. But the other side of the picture shows that contained in man's ability to perceive the future or to feel into it there are also the capacity to experience beforehand as a psychic foretaste the pleasant and joyous tones of life.

Mrs. Gogh wrote to tell me of her psychic experiences, describing those visions which enliven our thoughts about those that come from and retire into the unseen realms of existence. "I feel that I must write to you after your appeal in the press. I am a widow and lost my husband two-and-a-half years ago after forty years of married life. He is always so near to me and has appeared three times during the last three months. I woke one night and there to my surprise I saw him lying in the bed next to me. He disappeared as I spoke to him.

"On another occasion while awake I heard a scraping sound, and there he was sitting in his rocking chair cleaning his pipe with his knife. Again he disappeared when I spoke to him. Two weeks ago I woke with a pressure on my foot, I looked up and there he was standing at the foot-end of the bed smiling so sweetly at me. I was excited and said "Oh Dad" and again he vanished. I must add that my room is very light at night so I saw him quite plainly.

"In 1928 we were in England on a holiday and on the 19th December I was sitting in a room by myself and I heard my mother say: 'My girl don't cry for me I am happy.' I told my husband that I thought my mother had passed on. The next day we received a cablegram to the effect that she had died on the 19th December.

"Our son was a lad of eighteen when he went to war in 1939. One night I saw him sitting on my bed making dreadful faces as if in great pain and holding his leg. I called out to him asking what was wrong. My husband woke and spoke to me. I dropped off to sleep and then saw my son again, hopping right into our room on one leg. Again I called his name. My husband woke and asked me why I had called my son's name?

"I took notice of these dreams and believed that he had been wounded. For two weeks we had no news and then we heard that the Transvaal Scottish were cut up, and we received a wire that our son had been wounded in the leg. When he came home on leave he said that he thought of us—but he was light-headed, and thought his leg had been shot off; he came to himself hopping around on one leg. This was up North." Now his mother saw him hopping into her bedroom. It is quite possible that she saw an astral projection of her son at the time because his consciousness was clouded.

Mrs. Pieterse writing in Afrikaans described some interesting para-psychological manifestations.

"I am one of those people who see coming events and have had precognitive experiences since my childhood years. I see these things so frequently that I consider them as part of the normal function of my mind. Many of these I understand immediately but others have a complex symbolism which I cannot explain.

"For instance the simple ones concern illnesses and births. I have precognitive impressions, sometimes weeks beforehand. But most of my experiences of this nature are visions of events. I see them in broad daylight as they displace what else I am looking at, and the vision is as clear and life-like as a cinema film. I have seen horse races being run hundreds of miles away. I want to impress upon you that I do not dream these things, and I have no dream experiences of a precognitive nature at all. In these visions the events are taking place in broad daylight just as they happen weeks or months later.

"Some years ago someone whom I knew well, who has since died, decided he was going to buy some diamonds from the illicit dealers. When I was told in secret about his plans I warned him because at that moment I saw a native man standing in a hole in the ground; he had some front teeth missing and I knew he was a trap. In spite of my warnings my friend nevertheless went to do the deal. He was directed to a native whom he found standing in a hole in the ground. He told the native to open his mouth and there he saw several of his front teeth missing. At that moment he thought of my warning and the correct description of the native so he left the diamond buying alone.

"I have had many other experiences but I thought that this practical one of an attempt at illicit diamond buying seen a few weeks before the time would interest you. I have frequently seen the apparitions of departed ones. These spirits come to visit the farm where I stay, and there is one who is often with me and seems to want to communicate something to me, I am a little nervous about this but I don't mind seeing the visions."

Sister Perold writing in concise Afrikaans described her psychic faculties from the age of six.

"My late father was a great musician with the concertina, and I used to sit flat on the ground between his legs while he played the concertina above my head. My thoughts used to take wing when I listened to his playing of the lovely melodies and old-fashioned Boer music that stirred me.

"Then one day sitting in my usual place flat on the floor between his legs I was entranced by his music, when suddenly I saw a vision as clear as anything right before me. I saw water and on the water her face and her little 'kappie' appearing above the surface of the water was my little sister. I gave one scream and ran like the wind. I ran straight into the dam which was about fifty yards from the house.

"We were indoors when I saw the vision. My mother and father, surprised beyond understanding at my behaviour ran after me. I plunged into the dam, just as my father grabbed both my little sister and I. She fortunately survived but was nearly drowned. Afterwards we learned that she had followed the little ducklings, wanting to catch them and got into deep water.

"On another occasion I was lying on my bed, yet quite a little girl, when all of a sudden I saw a clear vision of the huge pot in which we cooked our farm soap. I saw the handle of the ladle which was used for stirring the soap, also the flames leaping up around the pot and the bubbling boiling soap inside. Then I saw how my little cousin of eighteen months climbed up on a little bench next to the soap pot and how she peered in, take the handle in her little hand and then she just tumbled into the pot. I screamed, jumped off my bed and got hold of my aunt's dress attempting to drag her out of the house towards the boiling soap pot.

"I shouted : 'Baba has fallen into the boiling soap,'but she laughed and said: 'No she is asleep under the tree." I ignored her and ran screaming, beside myself with distress and my utter helpless state, knowing that an awful tragedy had taken place. When I got outside there was no baby under the tree. This time my screaming was so piercing and terrorstricken that my aunt came running out to find the baby no longer under the tree.

She looked at me as if stunned and I could not speak. All I could do was to point at the soap pot. They took out the remains, because the caustic soda or whatever it was that was in the soap had destroyed the body.

"I can relate many of these experiences wherein I see future events as clearly as if I am watching a cinema show." Sister Perold's visions of course were not precognitive, they took place almost at the same time as the tragedies. But the impressive salient point is the fact that man's mind is capable of seeing an accident or happening at the time that it is taking place without the use of normal eyesight.

This inner sight is not obstructed by walls or any material physical barrier to sight. It seems to be taking place on a plane transcendent to the vibrations of the physical world of sense impressions. If events in this world of sense, and physical reality are reflected on the astral plane then one can imagine that Sister Perold's astral self was seeing what was happening on earth in the mirror of the astral.

The precognitive vision of Mrs. Pieterse, where she saw the native man standing in a hole with his front teeth missing, weeks before the actual event on this plane, must logically leave the impression on one's mind that the event was already in existence on some plane antecedent to this physical world.

The philosophical significance of a reality that completely ignores our time and space does indeed show the limitations which have been imposed on man by his brain. It seems as if this organ concentrates consciousness into a few meagre channels of knowing, and that transcendent to it lie psychic faculties capable of a vast expanse confluent with a cosmic consciousness.

These simultaneous clairvoyant visions which at the same moment perceive the event as it is taking place, clearly indicate a channel of perception revealing some of the hidden natures of the human personality. No doubt in most of us these faculties are dormant because we predominantly employ our sense organs, but my correspondents have emphatically shown that there are numerous people, who as a result of the nature of the integrations and interassociations of these different wavebands of energy, constituting what we know as mind and body, have acquired the power to utilise these transcendent faculties of the astral personality. In consequence they are more sensitive than most people and at times it does appear as though this higher astral perception seeps through into normal consciousness.

There are erudite intellects who have expressed the opinion that these psychic phenomena and faculties are in reality relics of our ancestral primitivism. They are viewed, therefore as archaic and atavistic remains which are today anomalies in our evolutionary state of development as homo sapiens. My view is of course dramatically opposed to this conception of atavism. I consider these psychic phenomena as revelations of the higher qualities and functions of the human psyche. They are to me faculties of our higher selves at present dormant in a relative sense within our physical personalities. But owing to certain variations in the integration of our energy systems within the personality they at times slip through for constitutional causes and in spite of the limitations imposed upon us by our brains, they introduce us to other worlds of our beings. Indeed where little children reveal these hidden psychic functions we are confronted with little witnesses of a reality which cannot but otherwise be at home in the nature of man.

Mrs. B. who is a kindergarten teacher and who studied psychology for her profession at university wrote in Afrikaans about her little son Hennie. "When he was a little more than a year old, and could only say a few words such as Hadda for Daddy and Mamma doo doo he took seriously ill with a severe attack of bronchitis. My husband was working on the mines and he had to leave for an early shift, having sat up the whole night at the bedside of our little son.

"After he had left for work I started on my duties in the house, keeping a constant watch on my baby who was asleep. All I could see were his little nostrils dilating as he breathed with difficulty. It was exactly seven o'clock in the morning, and I was in the room watching him anxiously, when the child jumped up out of his sleep, sat straight up and shouted, Mamma, Mamma—Hadda—Mamma, Hadda, Hadda, and then fell back exhausted.

"I thought that he was confused or delirious from the fever, and so attached no other importance to this sudden and strange behaviour of such a sick small child. But half-an-hour later I received a message that my husband had been involved in a serious accident underground and had been removed to the mine hospital. The accident had happened at seven o'clock and it was seven o'clock exactly when my little boy screamed in such a startled manner as if he had witnessed something terrible.

"When Hennie was four years old he was playing in the garden one day and enjoying himself, very absorbed in some game. I was busy indoors with my household duties when at exactly eleven o'clock he came running and called out in a distressed voice, "Mamma a motor car has just run over my 'Oupa' (grandfather). Where will I get another 'Oupa?' At first I did not concern myself about it but he would not go back to play. He kept on hanging around me telling me that his 'Oupa' had been involved in an accident and that I must find out what had happened.

"I then 'phoned my father-in-law in Standerton, but they were all quite well. After that I 'phoned my own parents living in the Cape Province in the Karoo. Imagine my astonishment when my mother informed me that my stepfather had been knocked down by a motor car at eleven o'clock that morning, but luckily was not very seriously injured."

Here again at the moment that the accident occurred this little boy in the middle of an absorbing game, received a mental picture or a thought that his "Oupa" had been run over. Even when seriously ill and a little over a year old, the accident of his father was at the same time perceived by him. It does appear as though there exists a short circuit of mind which flashes its messages along these wavebands guided by ties of affection, friendship and interest.

Two sisters wrote to me in Afrikaans describing an amazing affinity of feeling and thought. They are married with grown-up families and the one is four years older than the other. When they were small the family noticed with great interest that if the one child was ill the other would also be indisposed. If the one had toothache then the other had toothache and even if they were miles apart visiting different people and one of them should become sick the other would complain of identical symptoms.

No matter what the physical discomfort the other would share it, as it were. They were still quite young when they discovered that they dreamed the same precognitive dreams. When grown-up and living miles apart they would somehow become aware of each other's troubles and worries which were always immediately confirmed by telephone. They also observed that even if not in each other's company, one would in conversation with strangers sooner or later mention the other's name.

Emotions of distress or anxiety brought about by precognitive experiences would be shared as if they were one and the same person. At times they would think of each other and transmit thoughts which they would afterwards verify by telephone. Both of these ladies have children who are psychic with the emphasis on premonitions involving anxiety and distress. The mental picture presented by these two correspondents suggests the identity of the dominant frequency rates of their minds. This identification could primarily be in the vibration rates of their auras.

CHAPTER VII

PSYCHIC PHENOMENA IN AMAXOSA CULTURE

The native medicine-men or witchdoctors as they are commonly known, are divided into several groups. These range from those who almost exclusively rely on psychic diagnosis to those who dig and sell herbs and form the largest share of the group accused of being charlatans and quacks.

This group of herbalists is often labelled by the amagqira class as the practitioners of witchcraft or sorcery. They catch evil spirits and do a trade in love potions, and not infrequently as one travels through the Ciskei or Transkei one comes across some of these men accompanied by a number of women who are said to be learning the art of finding the healing herbs.

The herbalists are known as the amaxhwele, and constitute the lowest rank of those who participate in the art of healing. Some of them are extremely good business men and have become wealthy even by western standards. When however they are not successful in their prescriptions the amagqira are consulted, and the latter form the real doctor class.

The amagqira also employ psychic means for diagnosis and treatment, such as clairvoyance and telepathy. These are called divination because of the ritualistic requirements on which the fees are based. The amagqira however are superseded by the highest class of diviners and these are known as the isanuses.

They form the head or highest level of the hierarchy of healing and are often known by the term amatola. In the Eastern Cape there is a range of mountains known as the Amatola, the mountain of the diviners. No doubt they foregathered there in years gone by for their secret initiation rites.

It is accepted that those who constitute the true amagqira and isanuse group, possess psychic faculties in varying degrees. The isanuses especially have impressed me with their mediumistic powers and most frequently with clairvoyance. During the time that I did field work for my book *Sex, Custom and Psychopathology* (A Study of South African Pagan Natives), I met and associated with several isanuses and was often quite astonished by their telepathic and clairvoyant abilities. They believed that these faculties are inborn and could only be cultivated if present in the person. In other words if the constitution permitted development.

It was during this period of my study of Amaxosa culture and its mental illnesses that I met and became friendly with Solomon Daba who was an igqira, but in many ways he could have been raised to the rank of an isanuse, since in my experience I found his spontaneous parapsychic powers most outstanding.

There is an exaltation associated with the isanuse class. They form the guardians of the mystic knowledge, as well as the contact with the ancestral spirits, and the amagqira look up to them and frequently consult them. The isanuse prescribes medicines, but he does not himself dig them or carry them about with him. He makes his diagnosis by means of his psychic faculties clairvoyantly or telepathically, and with regard to the latter I have known of cases where the isanuse diagnosed what the patients believed were their illnesses.

Telepathic impressions especially among the amagqira often run this risk of receiving the patient's morbid imaginations. The isanuses are usually venerable men, and they like all good psychic sensitives even in our culture are rare. If there is an isanuse in a district he usually resides near a chief's kraal. The outstanding isanuses are excellent clairvoyants, and I do believe from what the famous isanuse Xagalalegusha told me, that they practise astral travel in their sleep.

During his consultations the isanuse does not as a rule employ the same ritualistic procedure of the amagqira. These as we shall learn later consist of chanting, handclapping and the beating of the drum. It is known by the name of ukwombelela. The isanuse only participates in these forms of séance techniques when he is called into consultation by an igqira. On such occasions the ukuwombelela precede the announcements of the isanuse of his communications with the onomathotholo or guardian spirits. They describe the nature of the illness of the patient and the medicines required.

Once a person decides to become an igqira he is required to experience a psychic condition known as ukutwasa. This condition in no way differs in its genuine form from those mediumistic manifestations which people experience in the western and other cultures. Many histories of ukutwasa cases contain early precognitive dreams, telepathic impressions and sometimes clairvoyance.

The experiences of Mrs. Shearer for example when she first revealed her psychic powers closely resembled those experienced by amagqira. Both Solomon Daba and Xagalalegusha described a genuine ukutwasa as consisting of some of the following experiences, namely cataleptic states, dreams of visiting other places with clear memories of these visits on waking, as well as seeing visions of coming events, and at times hearing the voices of the ancestral spirits known as the izinyanya.

The state of ukutwasa is characterised on the whole by such phenomena as I have described. The faculty of clairaudience or hearing the voice of an ancestral spirit is apparently not a frequent experience. Dream travelling and conversation with spirits are by far the most common experience.

I was impressed by the isanuse Xagalalegusha (whose photograph I took and published) when he informed me that ukutwasa was the coming into being of the powers, whereby man could at times establish contact with those who have gone before, and who live in the world of the izinyanya. What impressed me was his self-assurance about this ultimate reality. It was as though Outa Jantjes spoke in another's guise.

But Xagalalegusha as well as Solomon Daba made it very clear to me that there are many who claim to have had ukutwasa experiences, and who consider that they have been called to become doctors and diviners. They said the amaxhwele encourage these beliefs whereas many of these ukutwasa cases were people who had lost their senses.

They did not deny that people could lose their senses as a result of witchcraft and evil medicines, but however these conditions might have been caused, they were mental illnesses and not genuine states of ukutwasa. It is of importance to note that these men did make a differential diagnosis and did not accept every case as genuine merely because the person described or claimed the characteristic and expected experiences.

During my investigations I came across many cases of schizophrenia and epileptics who claimed to have been ukutwasa. Relatives readily accepted these claims since these conditions were endowed with blessings rather than the malevolent influences of witchcraft magic. It is easy to understand how the traditional pattern of belief, deeply rooted in the mind and carrying with it the guardianship, protection and wisdom of the ancestral spirits, could well up during exalted moods, and also in hallucinations of hearing during the disturbance of brain function with its consequent psychological disorder of thought.

A schizophrenic patient or an epileptic in an exalted mood could hear voices, see visions, and feel omnipotent in mood elevation, and so live the pattern of traditional spiritistic belief that the experience is supernatural.

The voice so often calls him to the hills, where he would find the plant that could cure all ills, and give him the magic elixer of life, and thereby master all the evil powers of witchcraft.

This culture of course has its host of mythical creatures. The native mind however does not understand these as imaginary or fictitious. They are on the contrary real beings but dwellers in an invisible world and nevertheless intimately concerned with the life of man. One set of mythical beings who seem directly related to social conscience is the Abantubomlambo or the River People.

The following description of the rites associated with the Abantubomlambo is quoted from my book *Sex, Custom and Psychopathology* :—

"With many native doctors or diviners in training however the ukutwasa may be manifested by being called to the River ukubizelwa ngumlambo) by the River People. The doctor may stay for ten days or more with these people underneath the pools. This is where he is taught the secrets of the medicines and gains much wisdom about the hidden mysteries of life. When he returns after several days, with many roots, barks and other herbal medicines and claims to have been with the River People, they know that he has obtained much knowledge and is a wise man. He is not questioned about his sojourn 'neath the deep pools, for if this is revealed he will be called again and killed. Thus his mysterious training underneath the water remains sealed throughout his life. The people merely accept that he has been there because he displays the gift of looking into the future as well as bringing to light hidden things of the past, giving love-charms, healing the sick, telling where stray and stolen cattle may be, knowing the wishes and secrets in the minds of others and, above all, speaking to the departed ancestors. His sojourn with the mysterious River People is like a journey to a distant world, indeed to a treasure house of knowledge, and thus his reputation as a doctor or diviner is greatly enhanced.

So the Abantubomlambo serve the people of the land by giving knowledge and wisdom to those suitable persons who are to heal the sick and combat the evils of witchcraft. But as guardians of morality they also punish those who offend against the moral conscience of the tribe and from time to time demand a sacrifice for a life that should have been paid by a human being. For this reason they exercise a mysterious call, only heard by the animal or person concerned. This call can be responded to from long distances, and the animal or human being thus called will make straight for the deep pool and disappear from sight. The natives express no resentment that their valuable cattle may be called to the River. They rather view this as a form of sacrifice or substitute for a human life. Besides, gifts to the River People bring retribution in health and good crops. Natives often express surprise if a white man appears concerned over the death of an animal, because they reason that if the animal did not die, he might have lost one of his family.

In olden times an annual sacrifice was made to the River People. An ox was slaughtered and the meat thrown into the pool.

This practice was then more explicit in appeasing the Abantubomlambo. The fear of their wrath was always to the fore. This is no doubt due to the advent of European law, magistrates and mounted police, as well as the host of educational influences from church and school. But although the annual sacrifice has disappeared and a sacrifice is made today only when someone has to be recalled from the River, this has in no way affected the vividness of the belief in the Abantubomlambo. The ceremony and sacrifice for recalling someone from the River People is performed under the direction of the chief diviner or isanuse.

When a member of a kraal appears listless, looks queer, roams aimlessly about, looks worried and anxious, ignores the questions addressed to him and fails to associate and communicate with those around, they know the power of the River People is at work and he may at any time be called to the River. He is kept under observation and soon, maybe, he will stand looking about as if in a dream and then start to run straight for the River. They call him by name, try to catch him and throw stones in front of him to distract his attention. They may catch him and tie him up at home until the Abantubomlambo have claimed some animal sacrifice as a substitute, but it happens at times that the one called will outstrip his pursuers and plunge straight into a deep pool. As soon as this happens they quickly return to the kraal to tell the others and to warn them not to weep, for if anyone weeps, he will surely be killed.

The isanuse is immediately called. He, with all the people of the kraal driving their cattle in front of them, proceeds to the pool. The cattle are driven into the pool and the one which goes farthest in is the one selected by the River People. This beast is slaughtered at the side of the pool, the flesh is cut into sections and thrown into the water. The flesh from the right side of the beast, they say, will remain in the water and that from the left side will float to the side of the pool. This is picked up because it indicates that the River People find the meat pleasant and have returned some. Should the relatives have no cattle of their own they must purchase an animal which must be fawn in colour. This has reference to the Hippopotami, which are considered to be the cattle of the River People.

From the time the cattle for selection are driven into the water, the members of the kraal gather on the banks of the river. With rhythmic clapping of hands a dance starts. A circle is formed and the dancers leap into the circle with stamping and prancing movements. The legs are thrown forward and brought down in an arched manner. The toes hit the ground first and this is followed by two jerky movements of the ankle and finished by a quick tap of the heel on the ground. The clapping of hands and the chanting grows in force as the dance proceeds.

The uninitiated, or those who have not gone through the Abakweta ceremony, press close together in a long single file. Their bodies pressed together, they stamp and chant; every now and then a flash and a clash as the kieries (sticks) meet above their heads. The dance continues, and, if the River People are satisfied, the one "called" will appear in the centre of the pool and soon after will emerge none the worse for his experience. He will then be taken in hand by the isanuse and treated for his abnormal condition.

The dancing and chanting may continue for days, and if the "called" one does not re-appear, it is a sign that someone in the crowd has wept and the River People have taken the life of the one they called. After a few days the body will be seen floating on the surface of the pool with bits of flesh bitten out. This, to the natives, is convincing evidence that he was killed by the River People. The presence of numerous crabs in these pools is in no way connected with the missing bits of flesh from the body.

It will be seen that the one who is called to the River People is mentally disturbed according to the description given to me, but the amagqira and isanuses equally claim that part of their training and preparation included a visit to the Abantubomlambo. There is of course a great difference between being called to receive punishment and being called to receive the gift of wisdom and supernormal mental powers.

It is indeed a great honour and privilege to have been taught by the Abantubomlambo. At first I was puzzled as to how the amagqira and isanuses could claim such a preposterous experience as a sojourn with the Abantubomlambo, and why they should accept and describe the literal interpretation of the rank and file as a veritable occurrence embodied in the sort of truth belief can fashion.

My intuition told me that the Abantubomlambo was a symbol and a rite representing a social conscience, and that its literal meaning as understood by the mass had not the same significance for the amagqira and isanuses. I sensed a mystery behind this story of a people who lived underneath water. The latter is a medium into which one can see but not live in physically, and if one could exist in it, the existence must differ from the physical above the water. The water hence appeared to me as indicating a supernatural form of existence for man, because in one's normal state death must follow such an existence. How could one breathe under the water without of course an apparatus which does not belong to this picture?

The association of the Abantubomlambo with the mediumistic experience of ukutwasa intrigued my mind. What was the real abstract symbolic significance of the Abantubomlambo? There was some particular aspect of mental life which the River People signified, but what was it? And then one day while in conversation with Solomon Daba and talking about the teachings of the Abakweta in their training for manhood, the revelation flashed into my mind.

I told Solomon Daba that his izinyanya had just told me the true meaning of the Abantubomlambo. He was amused and wanted to know what I had discovered. But as I told him my ideas on the matter his expression changed to one of amazement. I informed him that the Abantubomlambo were not physical people living under water. That was only a way of making people believe something that was good for them, but that the real truth was known to the amagqira and isanuses who held gatherings in places like the Amatola mountains.

I told him that the Abantubomlambo was a name for people who lived in a world, where sometimes they can be seen like objects can be seen when they come from the deep waters near to the surface. But that this was not a world for people of flesh and blood. It was a world where people lived who had left their bodies in the earth. It was a world you could visit in your dreams when your body is asleep. It was the world where the izinyanya dwelt. Therefore when one's mind went underneath the waters then it went where the izinyanya live, and there it would mix with their minds. In other words communicate with them and obtain wisdom from them. They live in a place where tomorrow is today because they could see there the past and the future.

Solomon sat and stared at me. Then he said : "So they have told you. Now you know that the water is the sky. The Abantubomlambo live beyond the sky, which separates their home from ours. You have found a great thing and it will not be difficult for me to teach you something else." On that particular evening we had some distance to walk from the kraal to where I had left my car. It was an evening of much beer drinking and the young bloods were roaming and looking for adventure. This worried Solomon who called me into his hut.

When we were alone he informed me that the young men who had been released from the Abakweta Lodges were a bit wild that evening, and he wanted to give me a sign for my protection. The Amatola had informed him that he could trust me with this sign, as I already knew it and its significance, although the Amaxosa words were slightly different. This sign was known to all natives initiated and instructed according to the traditonal rites in the

Abakweta Lodges. But it was not known to those merely circumcised in other places and in the hospitals of the white man.

He said the sign he was about to give me was as old as the hills. It is said that an ancient isanuse had received this sign from the amatola, when their remote forefathers had lived in a land of reeds. I interpreted this as the regions of the great rivers and lakes of Central Africa, before the southward migration of the Bantu peoples. He impressed on me the fact that this sign was to be used by me only on occasions when my life was threatened or in danger, and added "once you see it performed by me you will recognise it." He then stepped back and made the sign of "distress" as known in Scottish Freemasonry.

To return to the experience known as ukutwasa. The occurrence of these psychic states in a primitive culture, and the recognition that it is a mental faculty which all could possess, but few could develop is identical with conceptions which we have of such psychic phenomena in our western culture. It reveals powers of mind whereby channels of communications could be established with the ancestral spirits.

I have heard psychiatrists who considered that ukutwasa was a phase of the mental illness known as schizophrenia, and therefore in the absence of authentic information that such a psychic condition actually can occur in those not suffering from any mental illness, they have classified ukutwasa as a pathological state of mind.

My experience in this field gathered from isanuses and amagqira who have described their own experiences, as well as those of pupils who came to them for training and development of these faculties has left no doubt in my mind that the discovery of mediumistic qualities in this culture is always ritualistically dramatised and highly esteemed. Because since ancestral worship and appeasement are cardinal factors in the maintenance of self-preservation anyone with a faculty which can reach the people who live beyond the sky is a blessed asset to the kraal and the community.

The diagnosis of any mental pathology involving the hearing of voices as ukutwasa, is commonly made by the amaxhwele or herbalists. The treatment of these cases form a large proportion of their income. They readily diagnose a temporary loss of senses (to employ a literal translation of their idea of mental disorder) as the result of evil witchcraft effects, once the diagnosis of ukutwasa is not longer appropriate.

Patients who have been treated in this manner have often been seen by me in out-patient psychiatric clinics, and these patients usually came from large African townships in industrial cities. In these communities the amaxhwele swarm the healing profession, but they are not to be compared with the true psychic isanuse or igqira, who appeared to me to have something akin to an ethical standard for making the correct diagnosis. But where they diagnose a loss of senses or irrationality or any mental illness for that matter, they too fall back on the idea of the evil influence of witchcraft performed by someone as the cause of the illness.

Some examples of my experience of Solomon Daba's psychic powers as recorded in my book *Sex, Custom and Psychopathology* (A study of South African Pagan Natives) will reveal his amazing spontaneous ability to enter into what I consider is the astral mental dimensionality. I quote :

"I explained to Solomon Daba that I could not accept the numerous claims of supernormal powers made by him and his followers unless I could verify them for myself. He agreed to submit himself to any test I might wish to carry out. I therefore decided to bury an article on my next visit and test his powers for myself.

"Now Solomon Daba lives about sixty miles away from Queenstown. On leaving for his kraal, I buried in the ground a little cheap purse, wrapped in brown paper. Over the spot I placed a flat brown stone and on top of this a flat grey stone. Not a soul was in sight during this operation of burying the purse, nor did I, from the first moment the idea came to my mind, divulge my intention to anyone. From the moment I bought the purse, it was not seen by anyone, nor had anyone but myself any knowledge of the nature of the article to be used for this test. I left my assistant, Van der Merwe, in the car and went into the bush to bury the article. On leaving the spot, I travelled at an average speed of about thirty-five miles an hour. I mention this to obviate the possible explanation that he was informed by runners before my arrival.

"Shortly after my arrival I requested a seance dance and told him I had prepared a test. During the dance, Solomon Daba described in minute detail the article, the nature of the locality in which it was buried, the brown paper in which it was wrapped as well as the colour of the stones. During the dance I never once gave any information to show that he was on the right track. It will be assumed that he was reading my mind telepathically. I have no objection to this assumption. All I wish to add is that he accomplished a remarkable feat and displayed supernormal mental abilities. This is only one of many experiments in which Solomon Daba acquitted himself very well.

"A few months ago two cows were stolen, belonging to Mr. Victor, a charge nurse in the hospital. Shortly after this, I required

Solomon Daba's assistance in elucidating a few points on witchcraft and due to pressure of work in the hospital I could not find time to travel 120 miles there and back. So I requested him to come and see me at my expense. On such occasions, when I foot the bill, Solomon Daba takes a childish delight in travelling in hired motor cars. As a rule he occupies the rear seat alone and in state, with his monkey-skin headdress. Late in the afternoon, towards the close of our lengthy discussion on witchcraft, Mr. Victor entered my office. It suddenly occurred to me that this would be an ideal opportunity to test Solomon Daba's psychic powers. I informed him that I was going to test his psychic powers and merely added that Mr. Victor had lost some cows and asked him to describe the cows and give their present whereabouts. He said he would try, and there upon shut his eyes and sat quite still for a while. On opening his eyes he said, 'I see the cows and I know where they are and how they have been stolen,' and then proceeded as follows :

'There were two cows, both black and white, and the younger of the two was going to calve; in fact she has calved because there are three cattle now. The younger of the two cows has a peculiar mark on its left side, the hair has grown in the opposite direction in the form of a crown or whorl. There was a little white boy about six years old who was very fond of this cow. He always fed her with bits of grass and corn stalks. Late one evening the cows were driven away from the field by a native man who works in this hospital. He kept them at his house in the location that night and the following morning early he hired a native boy to drive these cows to a friend's place near Lady Frere (30 miles away). This boy left with the cows while it was still dark and drove them to the kraal near Lady Frere. He crossed the railway line this side of Essex and took a little-known track across the veld.'

"I, of course, could not verify his descriptions of the cows, never having seen them, but I doubted his statement about the little white boy since I was well aware that Victor had no such child. As instructed, none of the members of the staff present said a word.

"After Solomon Daba left, Mr. Victor corroborated his description of the cows to the minutest detail; even the doings of the little boy turned out to be correct—this was a neighbour's child. As the matter was already in the hands of the police nothing further was done. The suspected man went off sick a few days ago and while at his home sent a native boy with a note to the ward. Mr. Victor, having in mind what Solomon Daba told him, asked this native boy whether he drove some cows for X to Lady Frere some time ago. The boy, in my presence and that of other members of the staff and the police, admitted driving the cows and gave a description tallying in every detail with what Solomon Daba had said."

I attended several seances given by Solomon Daba and never found that he had fabricated a story. Always his predictions somehow came true. One unforgettable event was a seance especially given for my benefit on an August evening in 1936. It was one of those cold bleak days, and towards sunset the icy wind sweeping over the denuded hills and eroded dongas of the Ciskei penetrated its coldness right into one's bones.

The native people wrapped themselves snugly in their red blankets, and sought the inside of the huts, where many bodies and a central heap of glowing coals provided a drowsy warmth, and an atmosphere heavy with human exudations. There we were, a large number of men and women—we sat on our haunches around the wall of one of Solomon's biggest huts. Green mealies on the cob were being roasted and handed round to be washed down with long draughts of Bantu Beer.

These preliminaries included the melodious chanting accompanied by the clapping of hands, and so creating a regular succession of impulses, seductive in their blended effect on one's senses. We were waiting for Solomon Daba and his wife to make their appearance and to perform their famous seance dance to gain contact with the izinyanya. The chanting and the clapping of the hands had to provide the atmosphere of sound and feeling which would draw the ancestral spirits to our presence. Around the fire a narrow space was kept clear for the dancers because not much space is required to perform a dance of this nature.

The emphasis of movement is confined to groups of muscles accompanied by a stamping action of bringing the foot down on its front part with a quiver of the heel before it too hits the ground. Vibratory movements of shoulder muscles and buttocks in the case of women seem to give expression to an inner rhythmic emotional tension in which the power ripples along the arms and legs. My assistant Mr. P. van der Merwe was next to me and we sat with our backs against the wall and between us was a cannister of Bantu Beer.

Mr. van der Merwe grew up amongst these people and as a boy fought his way to expert standard as a stick fighter. He spoke Xosa in all its shades of meaning. Indeed their poetical thought stirred him with delight, and their feelings about their customs and values resonated among his sympathies.

He spoke Xosa with a musical lilt which never failed to draw exclamations of appreciation from those who were adept at the use of the idiom. He could enter so completely into the spirit of the language, that nothing in its meaningfulness escaped him.

He would thus fill in the gaps in my comprehension as the chanting and clapping were punctuated by some remark or expression of feelings. There was magic in that rhythmic stimulation of one's brain, and it slowly drew one's feelings closer and closer into a whirlpool of unwitting incantation. Every expression seemed meant to penetrate the veil between this world and that, and at the same time maintained a tempo of invocation casting a spell over thought and emotion.

The warm heavy atmosphere drove one from time to time to climb over seated bodies to fill the lungs with the cold air outside the hut. The native people laughed and said that soon I would prefer to be cosy rather than breathe cold wind. The Bantu beer added its quota to my mental heaviness, and increased the drowsiness which the melodious chanting cadence pulsated through my being with the tom-tom metre of the cow-hide drum.

Near the door sat a number of women, and before them was a curled-up dried cow-hide skin in the shape of a roll of linoleum. As they chanted, while others clapped hands, these women produced a rhythmic thud, thud, thud beat with short sticks on the cow-hide. For almost an hour-and-a-half this lulling rhythm of hypnotic potentialities went on and on preparing our moods and harmonising our thoughts into one eternal direction. The voices from time to time would rise vibrant and clear in their appeal in words—"Come ancestors and make these things clear to our understanding."

This power of the pagan soul stood naked before me in its primeval religion with its mass consciousness to reach by means of feeling those who have gone before, and who knew today what unborn tomorrow would bring forth; for they did not move with the rising and the setting of the sun, their days and times were different, for to their eyes there were no nights or days, no barriers through which their minds could not penetrate. After a time one began to blend with this weird and fascinating spirit, while its alluring power seemed to resonate the rhythmic pulse of all of one's being.

At last Solomon and his stout wife appeared and as they entered they danced. The choral music which was played on a gramophone before the Scottish landlady went into a trance had its equivalent in this expression of rhythm. There appeared to be a need, some unfathomable relation between rhythm or vibration giving ease of self-expression, and this aspiration for a deeper self to come to the surface.

Somehow this rhythmic, melodious tempo, this unison of all feeling, and this singularity of thought's purpose, hearkened back to some archaic awakening, whence consciousness could rise unfettered by the trivialities of this world and its business of living. When Solomon began to dance every movement, every beat, and measure of handclap and chant formed one flowing stream of motion in which all took part as imagination conducted this orchestra of emotional intunement.

His powerful arms were covered with rows upon rows of brass bangles. From his neck over his chest hung several closely beaded necklaces, almost identical with the pattern which one has so often seen in pictures around the necks of ancient Egyptian rulers. I was amused to observe that he wore his famous kilt which reached just above his knees. This garment he always wore when he came to visit me in Queenstown. It was beautifully ornamented with brass and beadwork.

As he danced he swayed his hips which gave a swagger to the kilt. He was an impressive and powerful man and wore around his head a beaded head-band from which dangled short strings of beads giving a tasselled appearance. On his head he wore a cap or head-gear made of the soft furry skin of the monkey, the tail of which hung down the back of his neck. His wife was a very pleasant person and she too wore a monkey skin head-dress, while her skirt was richly adorned with intricate patterns of bead-work. Her mediumistic powers were well-known and she acted as her husband's assistant.

I was impressed by a characteristic repetition of one particular movement or posture in his dance. Time and again his dance would stop and he would be poised in an attitude of supplication. His hands, palms upwards and fingers cupped would be outstretched, as if asking for alms, as though receptivity was the soul of all his actions. Then again the movements of the muscles, their vibratory quivering would portray an ecstatic mood; as if he were aware of the proximity of exalted beings.

Nevertheless I could not help but believe that all his actions, the chanting, the beating of the cow-hide drum, the voices of appeal to the ancestral spirits—all symbolised an imploring attitude even the entreating gestures of the open palms, and extended hands were gestures which beseeched the izinyanya; all were embodied in the chorus which swelled into "Come ancestors and make these things clear to us."

How could one exclude a religious feeling from all this transcendant aspiration of primitive hearts? I asked myself whether the feeling of one's being had to reach a certain pitch for the field of force to become the expanded receiving consciousness of thoughts from beyond the grave? There was a steady increase in the electrified atmosphere of mind for as the pulsations of song, chant and drum swelled louder and louder the call of the rhythmic soul became irresistible and others in ecstatic mood flung themselves into the dance in that small space around the glowing coals and roasting mealie cobs.

The mood of ecstasy was the dominant tone, and was symbolised and expressed by the extended arms in winged attitudes of flight, with bodies poised on the tip of the toes to represent the inarticulate patterns of soaring emotions and meanings. By means of the dance they were praying and in movement of ritualistic rhythm they were attempting to reach beyond themselves. Such is the primitive picture of man's soul in quest of higher expression.

The dance went on the hours went by and the sun had set. Time did not matter, and there was no hurry. We live now and tomorrow takes care of itself. Once could not command. The spirits had their own way of answering a call. One could only appeal, supplicate and dance and be patient, for their time was their own. As Solomon danced one could feel the vital fervour, the elated mood, and the power inherent in the traditional appeal of the dance. Even the thud, thud of the cow-hide drum in harmony with the beat of the chanting, and the punctuation of the clapping hands, all swept one's mind onwards dreaming with the passage of life, and the tempo of strange emotions.

My thoughts travelled to England. I saw my book being reviewed by Professor Seligman. I was going over to spend the Christmas in London. In my day-dream I met all my old friends, visited theatres and generally enjoyed a white Christmas in England. I had decided to take my manuscript over myself and to have a vacation and a sea voyage. My arrangements were already under way and so wrapped up mentally in this peculiar lullaby atmosphere and its influence my imagination roamed about London and Oxford.

Then I was brought back to earth by a nudge from Van der Merwe. The ancestral spirits were coming through and the first chorus of "Siyavuma" meaning "We agree" filled the hut. I listened and while Solomon talked Van der Merwe helped my comprehension by a whispered translation from the Xosa into Afrikaans. Now would come revelation of the hidden things. All was silence. The dance had stopped and Solomon began the communications of the thoughts which he received from the izinyanya.

At the end of a certain number of ideas he would shout in a booming voice "Siyavuma" and all present would echo as one, "Siyavuma" and end the word with a simultaneous clap of all hands. Solomon Daba turned to me and said these thoughts have travelled through the skies of another world, they concerned me. He said that I was thinking of going over the huge ocean in a big ship to a land with many houses and much smoke, where the skies were dirty and the clouds not as white as ours and where the stars seemed to be without light. I was going there.

At least these were the thoughts that were hanging around my head. I was thinking of warm houses, warm fires, many friends and snow like the fleece of the lamb falling all over making all things dirty appear clean and white. I was thinking of going before Christmas so that I could talk to other men about my book, and things which I had seen and learned about the Amaxosa people. But all these things which I have dreamed that day will not happen in that time nor in that manner.

Because he has received word from the izinyanya about the future. I would take ill, my throat would become very painful, and I would have to go to hospital where a doctor with dark-rimmed glasses would attend to me. Then after leaving the hospital I would be weak, and a friend who lived high up in a mountainous country with many fruit trees would invite me to recuperate on his farm.

He than went on to describe this friend as a man who used to sail the seas, and had two rows of brass buttons on his jacket. He was shortish and stout. I would stay up there among the high mountains and every day when the sun was near the middle of heaven my friend would open a bottle of bubbling wine and we would drink this to make me strong. Then after a while I would take another ship and sail over the seas to arrive in England the last day of March 1937.

At the end of the "Siyavuma" I said to Van der Merwe that I thought this time Solomon had drawn on his imagination. I paid little heed to his prediction and went on to complete my arrangements. I was determined to reach London just before Christmas. Then when it came near the time for my departure I developed a sore throat, and within a few days had a double quinsy. I could hardly swallow and felt very ill. My colleague Dr. J. M. van Schalkwyk decided to remove me to the Frontier Hospital in Queenstown. He wore dark horn-rimmed glasses.

When I left the hospital I received a letter from my old friend Commander Thomas of Elgin in the Cape. They wanted me to recuperate on their lovely and famous apple farm, snuggled among the forests and gigantic mountains of the Western Cape. Solomon Daba's description of Commander Thomas was almost photographic. There during those balmy days of the Elgin summer I soon began to regain my vigour of spirit and body. But every day about noon my friend would open a bottle of South African sparkling wine and among other things we drank Solomon Daba's health.

At last I obtained a berth and landed in England on the last day of March 1937. The white Christmas had turned to fog and slush. Solomon Daba during his seance dance firstly described what I was thinking, and I must add that I had not discussed my plans with him at any time before or after that seance.

During his description of my thoughts and my intentions he informed all of us of what I had been thinking during his dancing. This was then a concise and clear example of telepathy. But then he proceeded to describe what was going to happen to me. He also gave a description of Commander Thomas of whom I was not thinking at the time. His precognitive visions all came true. They unfolded themselves in a most amazing manner including the drinking of the wine at noon, and the stepping ashore in England on the last day of March 1937.

Solomon had told me on previous occasions that the information did not come all at once. It came in dribs and drabs. He would dance for a time, and then stop and relate something and then dance again to receive some more information. The whole process of communication hence could take quite some time. This ability to prophesy, to predict and to describe events in the far distant future coupled with telepathic forms of mental contact seem to be the most common among the amagqira and isanuses.

The problems about which these people are consulted concern in the first place illnesses, with a ready-made expectation in the patient's mind that some evilly intended harm had befallen him. The habitual attitude of the witchdoctor is therefore to gain impressions and often he merely tells the patient what are already fears or suspicions in the patient's mind. The ritualistic methods would then be employed and since there is always some dread that the person might have neglected to carry out some rite after the death of a parent to appease his soul, an illness could be bad luck or the result of his having neglected to follow the expected custom.

Lost property, strayed and stolen cattle constitute another important aspect on which the amagqira are consulted. These matters demand clairvoyant, precognitive and telepathic psychic faculties. It is of interest to note the spiritistic difference between the pagan medium and the one reared in western culture. Solomon Daba seldom gave me the impression that he was receiving his ideas from a single individual or spirit entity.

His communications and the manner in which those present in a séance behaved suggested that he was contacting a sort of hierarchy of wisdom, a celestial group-mind. Those who undertook journeys or wanted to make sure that their enterprises carried the approval of the ancestral spirits frequently consulted men like Solomon Daba but had to pay his fee.

Very often an article belonging to the person is requested and I have listened to some extraordinarily accurate descriptions of persons whose small articles I handed to Solomon Daba. We can then accept that psychometric interpretations are also employed to obtain information about persons, their characters or feelings towards the person concerned.

Forms of mediumistic trance such as is common in white circles, where the medium enters a trance and is controlled by some discarnate spirit seemed to be quite foreign to the pagan psychic phenomena and supernormal manifestations. The seances mostly consist of dancing such as I have described with the clapping of hands and chanting, while the medium remains fully conscious and describes the thoughts as coming into his mind.

It is assumed of course that these thoughts come from this hierarchy of ancestral spirits. I have seen Solomon in a state of mind which could be explained as trance-like. But this state did not comply with the true condition of trance because he was conscious and yet detached. He chewed some root and his eyes were fixed on some distant object with a sort of glazed look as if at that moment he were looking into some other world.

On other occasions he chewed a root and closed his eyes and during this period would sit absolutely still for some minutes, and when he opened his eyes he would describe the vision which he had seen as in the case of Mr. Victor's cows. But the vision could also be one that still lies in the far-flung future. One is of course always suspicious when people describe your enemies, or someone who would do you harm. One has learned to ignore these fortune-telling paranoidal ideas.

Yet one day on a visit to Solomon's kraal I handed him a box of matches to light his cheroot which I had brought him. He handled the box and said "This is not your matches, you put it in your pocket by mistake. This box belongs to a man who is going to cause you a great deal of mischief." He then gave a description of the person concerned, who was immediately recognised by Van der Merwe and me. Solomon was quite correct about the unnecessary unpleasantness which this man's petty-mindedness caused me. But Solomon also added that this mischief was necessary to make me come to a certain decision. Even here he was quite correct.

The dance with "ukwombelela" that is chanting and hand-clapping does seem to produce the highest degree of exaltation.

I could always observe an element of emotional uplift, a pleasure to serve and receive inspiration, and of course there must have been an enhancement of personality, and the feelings which linked the expectations with the supernatural. The "Siyavuma" showed the blend of emotions, the feeling of oneness and the traversing of the psychic distance to make the higher contacts with the izinyanya.

He once told me that when he chewed the bark or roots, or when he danced to the "ukuwombelela" he found himself farther away from the things and people immediately around him. He would think with those who knew the past and the future. On some of those occasions his mind became quiet and light. He did not think with effort as he normally did, because the thoughts came to him like the wind blows towards and against one. He conveyed the impression of a passive mental capacity to which ideas came.

The faculty of precognitive perception is one of which I have had a great deal of authentic evidence in the form of letters from people telling me of experiences. But the most dramatic and clearly descriptive narrative was that prediction concerning my illness and all the subsequent events. They followed in a natural order as foreseen by Solomon at least from five to seven months before the time of their material occurrence as physical events.

Evidence of this nature need only occur once to convey a significance, which completely transcends any intelligent scepticism which the most educated mind can advance. The question arises, from where did Solomon Daba obtain the information about events which only materialized up to seven months later? Surely his imagination could not have framed such a correct sequence, and this in contrast to all my wishful thinking, which he knew, and read as my thoughts, and then contradicted by a prophetic pronouncement.

How could events which had not yet happened in our world of time and space and matter be in existence? In whose mind are they housed? Because at the time when they were predicted by Solomon Daba they were images and ideas. They belonged to a psychic world and were the materials of that world. It is reasonable apart from being logical to accept that somewhere, somehow at that seance dance in August 1936 there existed in a psychic form the events through which I had to live.

When I told my friends in London about this particular prediction, they realized how seriously ill-equipped were our modern and educated intellects to reason about such profundities. It is always so much less challenging and disturbing to one's peace of mind to ignore them. But to me it is a challenge which must be accepted since it has presented itself to every generation in every culture since the beginning of man. It is a challenge to man's higher intellect and was always meant to take priority over a trip to the moon or Mars.

In the end which will be the most profitable to man, rocket travel to the moon or psychic travel to the source of thought emerging from an unfathomable cosmic consciousness? Somehow Solomon Daba's mind was carried away on the rhythm of the "ukwombelela" and in its expansion to other levels of consciousness it perceived the future in that world in the guise of an ever-present, and not a vague nascent experience of uncertain existence. Even the wine was seen to sparkle seven months before the event.

Surely these ideas which he perceived months before had existence long before they became my feelings, sensations and memories? In whom did they exist? Surely not in his mind as we know mind in our psychological conceptions? He had no power, as I have no power to create events for others to live and so compel them to individual experience? If on the other hand he received these ideas from his ancestral spirits, they themselves must have had mental access to this world of the future or have shared the consciousness which harboured these ideas and images?

It seems to me our reasonable deductions must accept this strange logic of supernormal contact and must agree that before I lived through those predictions of Solomon Daba's, they were realities in the cosmos. But where? in whom? and how? They were not fashioned by spirits for spirits surely cannot create a future for man? If the spiritistic conception is accepted and it is believed that Solomon received this remarkable prediction concerning myself from his ancestral spirits then they in turn must have entered a plane of perception wherein the nascent future was already revealed to the consciousness of spirit beings.

Precognition has therefore a tremendous significance for man's thought, especially his religious, philosophical and psychological thinking. We are led to conclude from its existence and its authenticity that the individual has a particular place in the sphere of things, and that his life has a mental future, whose existence, or at times mere glimpses of such an existence could be ascertained. The prophetic vision of Solomon Daba and the untold numbers of other people who have made predictions of similar importance, bear witness that within man's mind is a degree of consciousness, which can reach far beyond this humble world of space, time and matter.

It is not dependent on the erudite knowledge of a pragmatic world. It needs no science and no literacy. It just opens its psychic petals and vision has before it the core of things. These contacts of my mind with higher planes of thought in an environment of necessity laden with commonsense, seem to tell me that the individual moves forward in time as part of a psychic process of "Becoming".

Precognition should be hailed by all intelligent men and women as evidence of a psychic substantiality, for at times it seems to rise in regal disdain above our plans and schemes and would stir our fear as that vital instrument of self-preservation. In this frame of mind it makes us listen to a thought-world not spoken by the men and women around us. Robbie Burns must have peeped beyond this plane when he wrote "the best laid schemes o mice an men gang aft agley."

But the world from which comes the ideas, the thoughts which make up the precognitive picture are not inanimate pictures of things. They pulsate with life. They are thoughts of a dynamic nature. They concern a purpose for the individual. The latter is therefore not a mere product of a physical body with its temperament and characteristics, but it already has its life-span made so important as to have a record of the process of its evolution far beyond the reach of man's sensory world.

We are driven to accept that the mind which predicts correctly obtains this knowledge from somewhere outside its immediate consciousness. And always as in my personal experiences there is an element of strangeness, as though a portion of one's psychic being had vibrated on some higher plane. One is made to think of terraces of different frequencies and dimensionalities ascending in terms of consciousness into a vast Cosmic Self.

But this idea of postulating a Cosmic Consciousness or even a Cosmic Being who possesses the future, the present and the past will to many appear as far too simple an explanation. There are those who firmly believe that man's spirit transcending the physical self is the agent that creates its own future, but leaves a limited portion of the sensory mind with which it gropes its way through life.

This idea of one's life and its power to experience precognition, as a product of one's own spiritual creation does not appeal to my intelligence. It gives a sense of omnipotence to one's spirit, and an independent status, which is sadly lacking in the modicum of wisdom which it vouchsafes to its physical brain and its intelligence during earth life. I am more inclined to accept that the knowledge of one's future is in existence within a Cosmic Consciousness.

Perhaps each individual on earth is a unit within the Being of some Infinite Organism. I say infinite because as a mere part of the whole one is quite incapable of forming an idea of the whole.

But the psychic phenomena of our experience do show that each of us is endowed with different levels of consciousness, the lowest and narrowest rung of which is found in the physical being, as expression by means of brain.

The other psychic functions could almost be considered as dormant relative to our commonsense existence, and their growth might be dependent on motivations for the aspiration of thought. Some degrees of consciousness might awaken on this side of the grave and others long after one's sojourn on the astral plane.

Each consciousness expresses an Ego which adapts itself to the plane of existence. Whether it develops during physical life, or on the astral plane, when severed completely from the physical body, will affect its adaptation because it is natural to have a reactive reciprocity with its surroundings and state of existence. Its habits of thought and its excursions of thought into the realms of man's spiritual values must add some dynamic force to the process of becoming a more enlightened entity.

If therefore each individual is really a constituent of a Cosmic Being, and has as its destiny as an evolution within this Cosmic Being with the object of reaching greater and greater dimensions of consciousness concerned with the secrets of life, then it is reasonable to conclude that these psychic powers, which appear as supernormal to us in this life, such as clairvoyance, precognition and so on, are in reality germinal manifestation of the future faculties beyond the grave.

In some they are completely dormant as if non-existent, or merely embryonic, and in others they are more developed and more energetic and vital, as it were. In this latter psychic group as we commonly call these people, these manifestations are episodic, sporadic and seem to respond to a host of feelings, emotional needs and desires or some particular event having a special significance for that person.

Now it is my impression that these occurrences of a supernormal psychic nature are the result of an expansion of this inner or dormant consciousness into a burst of activity, which can as suddenly subside. But during this expansion it becomes active in a higher rate of vibration, and so coincides with one of the psychic planes of the Cosmic Consciousness. It is almost analogous to someone climbing a high tower, to be enabled to see beyond the rise to which his vision was previously limited.

This Cosmic Being or Infinite Organism as I have called it, could very well consist of space, matter and time as some of its attributes. Our Stellar System including our sun and its planets is known as a galaxy. Systems far beyond our galaxy are known as extragalactic nebulae. The astronomers have found limits to these

Stellar Systems, and what is more that these galaxies are in states of rotation.

Some of these stars seem to pulsate with light, and others show explosive phenomena like sudden releases of subatomic energy. Some of these gases thrown out by these stars have shown a velocity as great as two thousand miles per second. Could these constituents of space not be organs of a Cosmic Being? These are only the visible manifestations but our experience of psychic phenomena has produced a great deal of evidence of the existence of the invisible.

Is it not reasonable to assume that some all-embracing consciousness contains knowledge of all life units within its Being? And that each of these individual life units is primarily concerned with the preservation of its self as the fundamental quality of a differentiated life? If this conception comes anywhere near the truth we can understand why Solomon Daba was able to read my future, because somewhere in the Cosmos it was in existence.

It could of course be that his ancestral spirits acted as intermediaries, and relayed this knowledge to his mind. But they had nothing to do with my future, and therefore could not have been its creators. Even my own spirit, if it had planned my quinsy and the postponement of my trip, must have had a peculiar indifference to my material welfare, as well as my conscious mind, and even my active intuition.

This idea that we read our futures, or others do it for us from some Universal Mind seem to me to be in no way incompatible with man's God idea. Whether there are gods as a super race of galactic giants is a question which opens itself to speculation. But if I am able to reach a supernormal psychic experience, I do so to my mind by expanding my consciousness until it vibrates with the frequency of a plane of an Eternal Consciousness in which the life-line of my evolution is mapped.

This concept of being part of a universal whole, is well described in the Brahmin philosophy which states : "God alone is unity, all other forms of life as to their material properties are but manifestations of this unity in myriads of scintillations of his glory. God is both cause and the effect."

One can look upon man as an inverted pyramid whose apex is his mind limited by brain, biochemistry, temperament and genetic constitution, while the base rises into the dimness of thought which is the eternal future. I suppose each future is only perceptible for the plane of one's existence. But is this a predetermined future in which one moves as a pawn in the game, a robot of cosmic manufacture?

I am inclined to doubt such an eternal predetermined rigidity of life. Because the chief purpose of human life as I see it is to develop the potentialities of its consciousness and sense of values, as well as the attempt to comprehend the hidden significances which our senses present to our minds. In fact life seems to lay emphasis on the expansion of our mental worlds.

I must admit that neither Solomon Daba nor the isanuses had extended their thoughts and formed new ideas, and new curiosities about the powers which they found in themselves and others. They were harnessed by habit, ritual and tradition, and placed each foot in the same imprint made over hundreds of years. Mind was not unfettered in this respect, whatever might have been its abilities to imagine and phantasize other pleasantries. In its psychic world it was a prisoner of belief. It was chained to pagan dogma.

Perhaps there is a difference between the determinancy which we experience in a physical world as cause and effect and the life which we might lead on the next plane. The physicists discovered a law of indeterminancy when they studied the behaviour of the electron. They found that when light was allowed to fall on a substance electrons were emitted from that substance, but no matter how they increased the power and intensity of the light they could cause the emission of more electrons, but they could not increase the speed of the electrons.

Now the electron is an enigma, because it appears to be a charge of electricity without a body. Nevertheless it is still substantial. Why could there not be similar laws in the dimensions after death? Why could man's spirit not equally be a reality like an electron? Anyway, the physicists have found that when they employed a shorter wavelength of light, say a blue instead of a red light to fall on the substance, the electrons were immediately emitted at greater speeds.

I have previously advanced the idea that the evolution of life went into higher frequencies and shorter wavelengths of energy. My object in drawing an analogy between this idea and the behaviour of electrons could be interpreted to mean that life moves from long to shorter wavelengths and remain entities and individuals without material bodies as we know them.

I suppose in this life one has a universe of action, which contains the world of one's genetic or inherited potentialities. One is finite, and yet when we think in terms of consciousness and aura one is unbounded. The laws governing precognition would take the shortest distance between two points, and so give only the main essentials. But this universe of action could have deviating paths determined by certain needs for experience, which the inner consciousness requires for its development although this course may not suit the commonsense mind of the material world.

Now the blue-print of the individual's constitution contains those genes which provide the biochemical forces for his physical energy. His interests and drives as well as ability for abstract thought are determined by these factors including his temperament. In his universe of action many ideas, emotions and forces may coalesce to augment energy and others may rise in opposition from experience stimulating inhibiting feelings and emotions, and so prevent action in a certain direction. But finally the strongest and most powerful motive will prevail, to act or not to act.

The making and remaking of decisions may all be part of a process not yet understood by us. A process which then allows inner forces to group themselves and combine their energies until the most powerful motive decides the issue. The will is free to imagine, picture situations and consequences, wish and desire and in fact to sweep through a wide range of mental possibilities until the major energy channels become confluent for the dominant motive to action. But has this a connection with one's future?

The precognitive vision or thought contains the essence, as it were, of a myriad of thoughts, which belong to the world of indeterminancy, but the final issue is a determination brought about by constitution and mind-training. The Cosmic Consciousness could therefore contain a pictorial or idea-plane of the final outcome of the different human motive forces, within man's universe of action. But this does not imply that there is only one final outcome that had been predetermined. There might be several consequences depending on how the forces of the person's nature combine or are stimulated by hidden motivations from the astral self.

Even Solomon Daba told me that he had seen that if a person followed a certain course in life, he would meet with an accident, but if he changed his course he would escape it. In fact he has had precognitive experiences of more than one picture of motives. And yet the strongest motive does not always avoid the wrong course. Take my experience with the puffadder. I reasoned that I would find these snakes in the bushy parts and so avoided the reserve only to meet the snake in a place which I considered would be free of snakes.

It seemed that somehow it was inevitable for me to come face to face with the puffadder. The motive based on my reasoning for avoiding the snake made me nearly tread on it. Mentally I was detached and not observant. The general experience is that precognition is primarily concerned with anything that might adversely affect one's self-preservation or that of those whom you love. Even premonitions which occur more frequently than clear precognition, judging by the letters which I have received, merely causes a sense of warning not based on any objective information. There is an instinctive foreboding.

If one postulates a Cosmic Being embracing within its unbounded self all the heavenly bodies and all the life on other planets in our galaxy then one must credit it with a Cosmic Consciousness in which our psychic lives evolve and reach for their goals of enlightenment.

It seems reasonable for me to think that within such an All-Embracing Being there is a plane of "Becoming" in which are the ideas of unborn terrestrial experience. These could represent as its fundamental purpose the blue-print or life-lines for earthy evolution, and would thus reveal the process of inner psychic growth antedating materialization. It could be that man's astral consciousness actuated by emotions of self-preservation could have access to this plane of psychic blue-print and so produce precognition or premonition.

Irrespective of one's speculations about the cause of precognition and how these future events exist the fact remains that they must be in existence to be perceived in an extrasensory manner long before they occur in our physical lives. It is difficult in the face of facts of this nature to exclude the possibility of the existence of a psychic world which, in relation to this material existence, has something which is intimately connected with our actions and decisions and which has a mysterious antecedence to our material experiences.

Are there parallel lines in this Cosmic Consciousness in which thoughtforms vibrate with radiations sustaining our earth lives? We are impressed by the observable fact that man is born with strongly individualized psychic potentialities which respond to circumstances of life. There have been clairvoyants who have predicted the development of a child and the talents he would reveal which have come true years later. This to my mind is evidence in support of my theory that a genetic thoughtform serves as a blue-print of the ideal self.

The reason why I think that man has a universe of action, like a goat tethered to a pole—allowing it plenty of freedom within the range of the rope, is the interesting phenomena of the changes which occur in man. In psychotherapy one often sees how the ideal or true personality of the blue-print reveals itself with a more matured understanding of life.

Solomon Daba often gave me the impression of a double psychic personality. During the seances an inner astral personality took over in the guise of a subconscious intelligence with supernormal information at its disposal. But the emergencee of this knowledge into the world of words was almost like stuttering. This double psychic personality showed clearly its power to construct knowledge inaccessible to the brain and its sense equipment.

Even among the amagqira they have found that the ability to peep into the future or obtain ideas from the izinyanya is seriously hindered, if not stopped altogether, by violent passions, or serious worries. This faculty often varied according to the circumstances of life, hence it was frequently necessary to have the upliftment of the emotions by means of the chanting, handclapping and the beat of the drum. Then when the lightness came over him, he saw mental pictures and received the thoughts which explained them. He too was most amazed at the houses of London, the fog and smoke with its hurrying people.

The main channel of psychic communication of the Amaxosa is the land of dreams. Here too symbolic visual images play a prominent part. A dream of a deceased relative or father has always a significance which necessitates self-questioning to ascertain where in his ritualistic obligations some act had been neglected. Often these dreams are interpreted as forebodings of some misfortune and so invariably a sacrifice is made to appease Umdali (The Creator).

What has amazed me is that at no time did I come across a history of ectoplasmic production or materialization. There is of course nothing in this culture to encourage this type of mediumship. Actually I think it is unknown in the manner in which it has been studied by men of science and other renowned investigators of western culture. The pattern for psychic communication is commonly the actions required by the ritual and there is no unconscious trance state that I know of.

It could be that poltergeist type of movement of objects by invisible means often at the onset of ukutwasa might develop into ectoplasmic production if such a psychic sensitive is trained in a manner favourable for such manifestations. The psychic powers of the amagqira and the isanuses are chiefly those of telepathy, clairvoyance and precognition and the latter not infrequently is interpreted from dreams.

Certain evidence which came to my ears strongly suggested a projection of thoughtforms which appeared to the person concerned as a phantom. I am unable to exclude from my mind the possibility of this practice, as a form of witchcraft. If such a phantom could become entangled with the victim's aura could it not by these means drive him to suicide by drowning, which then becomes understood as a response to the call of the Abantubomlambo?

The existence of mythical creatures with mysterious powers of a supernatural nature in this pagan Amaxosa system of beliefs, makes it extremely easy for these creatures to be endowed with bewitching powers, including the power to materialize and assume various disguises. The three significant beings in the folklore of the Amaxosa are the Tikoloshe, the Impundulu and the Inyoka.

The best known outside this culture is the Tikoloshe, who is described as a mischievous little fellow with aggressive sexual proclivities. I know of cases of rape where the accused had claimed that he was possessed by the Tikoloshe. Most of the activities of the Tikoloshe are associated with females and when I questioned a large number of Amaxosa women on their knowledge of the Tikoloshe they spoke of him with shyness and a certain amount of embarrassment.

The picture that is given of him is that of a little dwarf but powerful in muscular development with sexual organs of an abnormal size. There are of course many Tikoloshes since they are said to have their own wives, kraals and way of life. They also live beneath the waters of the rivers and pools like the Abantubomlambo.

The Impundulu is a bird with long legs and a powerful carrier of witchcraft, and if not the most potent, then it is the outstandingly sadistic one of all mythical creatures. The Impundulu plays the most prominent part in persecutory bewitchment. It is the paranoid of the whole mythical creature world. Its kick causes one to cough up blood and tuberculosis is still known as the kick of the Impundulu. Another significant characteristic of the Impundulu is that he has numerous paramours and has sex relations with women in their sleep.

The Inyoka or snake is another of the mythical creatures. There are two kinds of Inyoka, the Ugatya is the charmed snake, and the Ingumbane is the evil snake. It used to be the custom and is still a practice for the elder women of the kraal to examine the girls to ascertain whether they have not had sex relations. These elder women who perform this function have told me that a mother who possesses a charmed snake hands it down to her daughter. Of course no one ever reveals the possession of an Inyoka.

There are certain forms of behaviour well known to the people which indicate that a woman is bewitched by a snake or keeps one for sexual purposes. Such a woman will lie abed, refuse to get up, laugh and talk to herself and appear to be secretly amused at something. I have seen many such cases who admitted the possession of the Inyoka. These were all cases of schizophrenia in Amaxosa women. Erotic stimulation by delusional imagery patterned on traditional belief provided the Inyoka. This charmed snake is harboured in the sex organ of the women and although it leaves her to roam and feed it will always return to the woman to whom it is attached by her desires.

I have made brief mention of several of these mythical thoughtforms, which people have claimed to have seen in the form of phantoms. I have dealt fully with this system of belief in my book *Sex, Custom and Psychopathology* (A Study of South Atrican Pagan Natives) but I did not enter into the possible role which these mythical beings might play in the world of extrasensory perception.

It is well-known that Tibetan magicians conjure up thoughtforms by the sheer power of concentration, and the faith that thought is a substance which can be moulded into shape or image. These thoughtforms were often created as companions, but they might just as well have been imbued with sadistic, aggressive and other qualities of an evil and antisocial nature. The magician might project his own malevolent repressions on to his thoughtform or phantom, and so live them out or act them out in the guise of another.

A mental process of this nature would still follow the fundamental mechanism of projection where man for instance projects his sexual and aggressive impulses on to others and exonerates himself.

Madam Alexandra David Neel had first-hand experience of this phantom formation by deliberate effort and for a particular purpose. Her experience seemed to convey the impression that once the thoughtform had condensed its energy into that of a phantom that could be seen it assumed other qualities which were contrary to what she wanted him to have and so became a nuisance to her.

This experience by an investigator of her calibre and status could mean that thought-being in the nature of an electromagnetic force would increase its electrical potential as it is being built-up into something definite. But all this power to my mind would be drawn from the field of force or aura of the magician or creative thinker making the phantom. Therefore when this phantom is completed it might be able to draw to itself some of the person's sadistic or aggressive or repressed sexual feelings and thus behave in a manner not originally intended.

The question to which I have never been able to find a satisfactory answer is whether witchdoctors in South Africa employ phantom formation such as observed by Madam Alexandra David Neel in Tibet? If our witchdoctors are occasionally capable of doing this, or have actually performed this feat of mind then we have an explanation for the common South African belief in "goelery." Could it also not account for those strange deaths where natives have gone into the veld determined to die, and have lain down and died without poisons or violence or any known disease?

Be this as it may there can be little doubt that the mythical creatures which roam the mental world of the Amaxosa culture were orginally thoughtforms created for a purpose, or as explanation for certain conditions, such as the erotic behaviour in certain forms of schizophrenia.

Perhaps these mythical phantoms in the folklore of these people were from the first the products of the mental process of projection. Man, as he grows up in any culture, must come across certain aspects of himself which he regards as unpleasant or dangerous. These he readily attributes to others, especially that which he condemns in himself, and even condemns vehemently in other people. His sexual and aggressive impulses are the common materials of his projection. In a delusional state projection makes it possible for others to fill his mind with obscenities and excite peculiar sensations in his body like the Tikoloshe, the Impundulu and the Inyoka.

If these mythical creatures, offspring of man's fundamental psychological projection mechanism, became traditional thoughtforms, they might under circumstances of concentrated mental intention in conjunction with the radiative aura of man, become phantoms which could be seen by some and so fulfill a persecutory role by invading the extrasensory perceptions of the victim. I am not sure but also not free of my suspicions that amagqira and amaxhwele do make attempts to create and send phantoms to carry out their intentions.

CHAPTER VIII

THE CHALLENGE OF ECTOPLASM

I wonder if any medical student has ever come across a text book on physiology or biochemistry that contained a reference to ectoplasm as a mysterious form of matter, which had been observed as an extrusion from the human body? It is therefore astonishing to say the least, that the disinterested curiosity of science has not been stimulated by the discovery of ectoplasm by men trained in scientific disciplines.

Medicine for example in its study of the functions, energies and contents of the living organism has so far in its view of the physical personality completely excluded from its considerations of living substance the evidence for the existence of ectoplasm as a constituent of the human organism. Medical science therefore gives us but a partial knowledge of man's true physical reality. But in saying that medicine has not penetrated to the physical reality of the human organism, I must add that medical truth is largely concerned with pragmatic matters—those that are convenient.

Nevertheless medical thought has advanced to levels of abstraction, which have equipped it to break through the barriers of gross physical perception, because daily our medical science presents us with a challenge for intellectual adventure. Perhaps many of us are influenced if not conditioned by the manner in which we are still being taught to think about things, for it does appear that we have abstracted certain aspects of nature by means of our scientific principles and observations, while others have remained meaningless, because of our inadequate frame-work of ideas about the nature of man.

I have often asked myself whether we can entirely exclude a subtle prejudice from this common attitude of science to supernormal manifestations? And candidly I think prejudice plays quite a definite role in determining this attitude towards psychic and supernormal physical phenomena, such as for instance the production of ectoplasm by a medium in a trance. This substance called ectoplasm or teleplasm has been studied by men of science over many many years, and yet no medical acceptance of its existence is acknowledged nor has any medical theory as to its purpose in life been advanced.

To understand this medical prejudice we must bear in mind the formidable role played by the evolution of medicine to free man's mind from the dark years of superstition and witchcraft.

Man's ignorance about this unknown magic which nevertheless was observed and experienced by him led to the rites of witchcraft and magical practices and beliefs which enslaved the sick and the mentally afflicted to the extent that the latter were burnt at the stake.

The history of psychiatry alone since 1795 is a monument to the spirit of human liberation from those who had confused the psychic phenomena, and the existence of the supernormal with mental illness, and in consequence proceeded to destroy the human personality to free it from the possessing devil. These ignorant practitioners and charlatans gave the world a distorted and untrue picture of the psychic phenomena of man. Some saw in them the powers of Satan. Others tried to claim them as magical assets for their own egotistical advantages as they do to this day. Therefore since medicine took the patient from their clutches, we cannot expect medicine not to be on guard against the falsehoods that could be propagated from these nebulous regions of mind.

Medicine hence requires new concepts in a new age, when even the fundamental electron as the smallest particle is no more and no less than a disembodied charge of energy. The mind is now faced with a universe of many dimensionalities, and it cannot continue to select only those characteristics which have for it a utilitarian significance, or which are easily understood by the commonsense mind.

We have reached a stage in the expansion of our universe of thought, when we must ask what is the significance of ectoplasm? where does it come from? and what is its function in the physical living body? It is known to be a quasi-organic substance which is extruded from certain mediums known as physical mediums when in trance. Generally this substance issues from the medium's mouth, as well as the eyes, the ears and the nose.

After leaving the body it can take various shapes, even those of faces, hands and whole human bodies. At first as it leaves the body or is extruded say from the nose or mouth it is in a vaporous state and from this sort of misty condition it quickly condenses to form a solid substance. The appearance even when in the substantial solid state may be just a mass and without any definite shape. But thereafter some positive moulding of this substance can take place forming objects, such as faces and hands and on occasions even complete human forms.

The ectoplasmic phenomena are always produced in total darkness. The experience of those who have investigated this physical manifestation is that light immediately disintegrates the ectoplasmic material and causes it to disappear. When we think of the reaction of the Scottish medium when the light was switched on during the levitation of the trumpet then we can assume that the power which moved the trumpet was of a higher frequency than the state of condensation in which it is perceived as a solid substance.

It has been found however that ectoplasmic forms and shapes could withstand the detrimental effect of flashlight photographs. This resistance is in all probability the result of the brief exposure to the light. It has been found that the forms have remained quite stable for periods, evidently not too long though under exposure to red light. Without photography we lacked the objective evidence which the scientific attitude demands. Fortunately photographic evidence of ectoplasmic productions is available and cannot be disputed as factual evidence.

My purpose in this chapter is to draw attention to the existence of such a living substance. I shall therefore draw extensively from the pioneers including such honoured names as Sir William Crookes who commenced his investigations in 1869 when thirty-seven years of age. He called these manifestations teleplasms and was a man renowned in the world of chemistry and physics. He took photographs and produced absolute proof of these extrusions and the formation of human forms which behaved as if alive, and then dissolved into nothing. As President of the British Association for the Advancement of Science he addressed scientists on this subject, and yet today science has remained as indifferent as it was in the days of Sir William Crookes.

Perhaps Sir William Crookes and the others I shall name had to prepare the way for an age of clearer and unprejudiced comprehension. It is necessary therefore when we are trying to understand these mysterious evanescent powers and manifestations of the human personality that we review the work of some of the pioneers. During 1935 I was working in the United States of America and there learned from a colleague of the experiments on ectoplasm conducted by the late Dr. Glen Hamilton, a Canadian surgeon who was also President of Manitoba Medical Association.

Dr. Glen Hamilton was an outstanding personality and quite apart from the prominent part he played in his profession including the post of lecturer in clinical surgery at his university, he was also an elder in his Kirk. My friend in U.S.A. had heard Dr. Hamilton lecture at medical congresses on these manifestations of ectoplasm and he also illustrated his lectures with slides. The profession listened to him with interest and respect but apparently the matter rested there. Somehow the medical mind could not see the significance.

In 1943 I read a review in the American Journal of Psychiatry of a book by a Dr. Glen Hamilton entitled *Intention and Survival* published by The Macmillan Company of Canada Limited, Toronto. My mind went back to the Medical Centre Broadway, New York and my friend's most interesting memories of Dr. Hamilton's lectures. He had died on the 7th April 1935. His son Mr. J. D. Hamilton published his late father's collection of records which were intended for that purpose before his death.

He mentions that the experimental room was kept completely dark except for the use of red light when it was necessary to have light. "Either before or shortly after the seance began cameras were opened without injury to the plates. They were left open until an exposure had been made or the seance was ended. This, added to the fact that flashlight was released by a push-button held in my hand, and connected to an electrical firing-device, make it possible to expose the plates at a moment's notice."

"But the question will arise how did we know where to focus the cameras, and in the second place when to release the flashlight? Astonishing as it may seem days, weeks, and sometimes months in advance we were informed by the leading trance entity (control) at what point the coming phenomena would in all likelihood appear. This might be on Mary's (the medium) face to the left or to the right, some spot within the cabinet, or a point close to the centre of the room. The trance directors as well arranged for and gave the signals for exploding the flashlight."

The mentioning of trance directors in the above quotation may be confusing to those not acquainted with the procedure adopted by Dr. Glen Hamilton. He discovered early on in his research of these extrusions of ectoplasm that there were psychic intelligences who claimed to be quite independent of the medium's personality. He was extremely hesitant and cautious as a medical man to accept the existence of these spirit intelligences who considered themselves essential and indispensable to the production of these ectoplasmic phenomena.

Evidently Dr. Hamilton was in a bit of a conflict for he did not readily want to accept that the spirits of departed ones were actually taking a hand in the production of this strange substance, while the medium was apparently unconscious of it all. One can imagine what went on in the mind of this medical man who was also an elder of his Kirk.

He found however that once he co-operated with these spiritual directors of the seance he obtained results. It is said that Dr. Baron von Schrenck-Notzing who was a psychiatrist also at first refused to accept the reality of the existence of spirit intelligences from another dimensionality and found to his dismay that he obtained no ectoplasmic manifestations, but when he agreed to co-operate with these spirit controls the manifestations were most successful.

Dr. Glen Hamilton decided that he should have "no a priori rejection of any aspect of the enquiry however bizarre or repellent they might seem." This was indeed a scientific attitude expressed in its conquest of the prejudice against the existence of man as a spirit being. He considered that the co-operation of his group with the trance directors as he called them was an essential attitude in the work underlying the entire investigation.

His training in the basic principles of science led him to concentrate on ectoplasm or teleplasm as he called it. He was apparently concerned just with the production of this substance, as an extrusion from the medium's body. He was fully acquainted with all the research in this field since 1869 by Sir William Crookes, and therefore wanted to re-establish and understand the biological significance of this mysterious substance without the assistance and participation of spirit controls.

His discovery that the acceptance of spirit participation was essential for the production of ectoplasmic manifestations in an objective and tangible form, opened to my way of thinking a far-reaching avenue of thought. Because it implied that a spirit intelligence was in a position to employ a certain frequency rate of energy which could extract, as it were, this substance from the medium's tissues and their cells.

To quote Dr. Hamilton : "These teleplasms brought to light a series of incidents which demanded the introduction of a rational intelligence which displayed what we shall call intentional activity. This intelligence in brief was very objective about the seemingly anomalous and incomprehensible teleplasm (ectoplasm). As this exceeded our understanding of the substance from every conceivable rational point of view, it clearly became necessary to make some assumption regarding the source of this intelligence. For these and other reasons the spiritistic hypothesis was chosen."

There were several mediums in Dr. Hamilton's group, but the one who produced most of the ectoplasm was a Mrs. Marshall, known in his book as Mary M. A word about Mrs. Marshall would not be out of place, for it at least would show that knowledge of this mysterious ectoplasm, which was proved by objective means was beyond her intellect and education.

In his book Dr. Hamilton gives her history as follows : "Mrs. Marshall is of mixed Scottish and Irish parentage and came to Winnipeg from Scotland with her husband and three children shortly after the First World War. Able to see and hear since childhood in a manner which she could not understand, she appears to have exhibited incipient mediumship all her life. Mrs.

Marshall, while having few educational advantages, is an intelligent and capable woman. She is well poised, cheerful with a healthy outlook on life and devoted to the interest of her family and her church (The United Church of Canada)."

Dr. Hamilton found that singing helped the medium to enter the trance state. There were no other means employed; no concentration. They sat and held hands as instructed by the spirit control named Walter, and then everything happened spontaneously. Walter especially requested the ten persons in the seance room to hold hands since this was "not only a contrafraudulent measure, but also, it was claimed, because it assisted in the production of teleplasm" (or ectoplasm).

They had previously conducted trance experiments with another medium called Elizabeth. She produced the movements of objects by invisible means, usually known as telekinesis. This particular research led him to establish the existence of an intelligence demonstrably independent of that of the medium. Then with Mrs. Marshall's advent both mediums saw and heard, clairvoyantly and clairaudiently the spirit director of the seances. "They said this entity was a fair, blue-eyed young man with a humorous mischievous temperament totally unlike any other psychic personality they had previously described. He gave the name Walter."

It is of particular interest when studying these trance personalities to observe that Mrs. Marshall over the course of years lost willingness to continue serving as a medium for the production of ectoplasm. She expressed her desire to withdraw from the work. It required a great deal of persuasion on the part of Dr. Hamilton to keep her attending regularly.

Her argument was that the sittings meant nothing to her apart from its scientific value to Dr. Hamilton. She had rarely any memory of what took place and she was not allowed access to the records of the seances. In fact each sitting was a period in her life for which there was no memory; besides she found them physically fatiguing.

This mental attitude on the part of the medium showed a decided lack of interest in the psychic research project, for at times it required the earnest appeals of all of them to make her consent to serve as a medium. Now what was of interest in this situation was that Walter added his appeals and persuasions while she was unconscious and in a deep trance. These were repeated to Mrs. Marshall afterwards and seemed to have had some effect on her reconsideration to continue as a medium, however reluctantly.

To me this experience was significant because Walter seemed

keen to continue with the experiments. His intentions and desires were to all appearances in complete opposition to the medium's normal self. It was Walter who suggested asking Mrs. Marshall's sister-in-law to join the group as a medium to assist her. In all respects Walter behaved as a personality whose mind and characteristics were entirely different from those of the mediums.

Walter made it clear that he had control of the source of the ectoplasms. At times psychic lights were seen in the seance, and he held himself responsible for these too. There was a box with a bell in it which was rung from time to time. The flash photographs showed a cord-like substance which extended from the medium's mouth to the electrical bell-box. The electric bell with one or more dry batteries was high above the medium's head against the wall. The bell circuit could only be closed by depressing an over-lid supported by a spring. The box required a pressure of one-ninth of a pound to depress the lid.

It was apparent that energy was drawn from all those who sat in the seances but the mediums were the main conductors and perhaps generators of this amazing form of energy. Furthermore the direct voice trance, the production of lights, the ringing of the bell by exerting force, and the result of flashlight photographs all had an enervating effect on the medium. I am quoting the following experiment from "Intention and Survival" by Dr. Glen Hamilton.

"Mary M. passed into trance, and in a few moments Walter came through using the automatic voice (The medium's voice). He said he could not expend his energy using the direct voice if we wished a picture. He gave us our choice. We decided in favour of a photograph, and the control said he would try. I then discussed with him the bell box signal. It was agreed that the control (Walter) would give six rings, then two, and I would take the photograph on a single ring following the signal. That is, I was to fire on the ninth ring.

"In a short time, the bell having given a few preliminary 'try outs' gave the six rings, at intervals of about three-quarters of a second. Then followed a pause of about ten seconds, then two rings, and again a pause of about ten seconds. Then came the ring for the flash. I allowed the ring to last about two seconds before the explosion, and it continued to ring for fully two seconds after.

"In this experiment I used four lenses : one quartz, one wide angle, and two Goerz stereo. The photographs shows the result ; a twisted teleplasmic mass of purest white attached to the left nostril and the left cheek of the medium, and extending well down to the shoulder level : a cord from the margin of the mass on the left cheek, leading straight to the corner of the bell-box nearest the medium. This cord appears to be dark in colour. In the picture taken with the quartz lens, it is visible for almost its entire reach up to the box. The glass lenses register the lower part of the cord fairly plainly and the upper part less so. Under magnification a second cord is visible.

"We noticed also that the bell rang during and after the flash; consequently the teleplasmic energy was sustained throughout. The medium was rather badly affected by this experiment; she reported to us subsequently that she had been very nervous and wakeful after returning home, and that she had vomited up some froth about two hours after the flash."

Here then the medium showed reactions of exhaustion, wakefulness and even nausea ending in vomiting up some froth. These reactions were similar to those experienced by the Scottish landlady in a trance after the lights were turned on. The energy was apparently driven back into the body and probably the main conducting area in such cases is the solar plexus. The strand or cord shown in Dr. Hamilton's photographs do bear a resemblance to what we saw in a flash extending from the landlady to the trumpet.

We have here evidence of the significant difference between light and darkness on the human organism under certain conditions. The fact that we seek darkness for sleep, and the theory that the astral body moves out of coincidence during sleep seems to suggest that darkness is associated with man's conservation of energy. In other words that darkness allows an interchange of energy to take place which is prevented in daylight.

The aura of man, or his field of force may be absorbing unknown radiations of cosmic energy during the night and in darkness, which is not possible in the presence of inhibiting white light or daylight. Night and day seem to hold a mysterious meaning for life, when looked at from this aspect of the behaviour of ectoplasm to light waves. I might be wrong, but I have always had the impression that people who work at night and sleep during daylight hours, never appeared really as vital and energetic as they did during a normal routine of sleep at night.

Dr. Hamilton observed a marked difference between the substance forming the bell cords and the non differentiated ectoplasm —that is where the ectoplasm is just an amorphous mass. He noticed something which were observed by other investigators namely that the white ectoplasm was composed of individual compactable fibres. This fibrous appearance of the ectoplasm bears a correspondence to the muscle fibre system of the body.

The bell cord was also of a thread-like substance, which extended according to him a distance of about four feet from the medium. He considered that the properties of these two manifestations were unrelated. But to my mind the difference is only in the use to which this type of energy in its condensed form is put. It is apparent that the mass of ectoplasm has threads or strands, there is hence no reason why these strands or threads could not be separated from the mass for certain purposes or manipulations.

It is evidently the same energy system which forms the astral cord or cable or the silver cord of the Bible. According to Sylvan Muldoon the thick cord with its strands near the body extends until at great distances it is a mere thread of a cobweb. Walter told Dr. Hamilton that he could use this energy system for the production of direct voice, and he could use it to produce ectoplasm. To employ the energy for both purposes would evidently use up too much power.

He mentioned however that he preferred the direct voice in spite of its consumation of power because it afforded him a mechanism for conveying his own ideas and thus express them uncoloured by the personality of the medium. If one assumes that during a deep trance the astral personality with its consciousness moves out of coincidence to permit a spirit-being to link up with its field of force, and so control the medium through the vital silver cord, then direct voice would imply a greater separation of the astral body of the medium, than would be the case with the automatic voice.

Dr. Hamilton produced an actual flashlight photograph of a mechanism under Walter's direction for the exercise of the direct voice. The substance seemed to have been organized into some bell shaped form and composed of numerous hair-like strands of dark material. It could be that these fibres produce vibrations under astral thought-control, and so bring about vocal sounds and articulation.

It is quite clear from these experiments and those of other investigators that ectoplasm or teleplasm is apparently self-luminous. This luminosity was found to vary. At times it would be of a dull glow and as seen by Dr. Hamilton increase in intensity until it appeared as a brightly illuminated watch dial. Dr. Hamilton thought it probable that the light issued from a flat disc-like formation at the end of some ectoplasmic extrusion from the medium's body.

When we consider the visions of the dead clearly seen by people as if they were self-luminescent, and also those balls of light of a premonitory nature mentioned by some of my correspondents, then we can assume that these lights and self-luminescence of beings were due to the presence of ectoplasm drawn from the person who saw these visions.

The question arises whether ectoplasm normally exists in the human organism in the manner in which it has appeared in photographs? Or whether the substance photographed as a white mass is a condensation of millions of delicate and normally invisible threads of energy forming some inner constituent of our bodies, and perhaps mainly concerned with the conduction or generation of bioelectric forces?

But it is all so extremely fascinating to know that these hidden powers are within us, and yet we to our knowledge have no conscious will-power control over this energy system. There must be a very good reason why spirit entities have employed their techniques to disintegrate or dislodge this inner energy system of man to produce it objectively as extrusions of a sort of gelatinous mass from parts of a medium's body.

Apparently it is not stubbornly bound and adherent to the tissues of a physical medium, as it is in relation to the tissues of the average person. It is something which is an undoubted vehicle of life forces. I shall give examples of such animations, but at this stage I am more concerned with the inner purpose of ectoplasm, or shall I say its physiological functions.

I have had an intuitive impression for years that ectoplasm plays a definite role in the healing of wounds, and other disease conditions. A little reflection will show how quite healthy people have wounds which under the best care take longer than usual to heal. How far is it possible for man's thoughts of a pathological nature to retard recovery from a physical disease because of the influence of thought and emotion on the ectoplasmic energy system? Perhaps it plays quite a prominent part in our so-called pyschosomatic illnesses.

But the fact that the production of ectoplasm from a medium is accomplished under the direction and control of a discarnate being or spirit being is a problem which needs interpretation. The existence of an astral personality, and the production of ectoplasm as an energy system capable of effecting physical manifestations, such as moving objects and ringing bells and so on, provides evidence that the human being is composed of many different systems of energy forming his spectrum of life.

From time to time we read of people who claim miraculous cures as a result of some unorthodox treatment, some sort of faith healing, like the people who claimed to have been healed at Lourdes, and others cured by consistent and persistent prayers, or some remedy advised by psychic means. A great deal of this evidence is usually so covered by emotional valuation that the physiological healing processes are attributed to miraculous intervention of supernatural power. But when one critically examines some of these testimonies of people, and the examples which they quote the conclusion is forced on one that it would be sheer prejudice to dismiss this unknown process of healing which responds to prayer and mediumistic psychic influences.

The evidence which I have quoted from the late Dr. Glen Hamilton's research leaves a very strong case for accepting an independent spirit intelligence operating by thought-power on a physical medium to produce ectoplasmic manifestations. I shall quote further evidence from the experiences of others in this field especially the classical work of outstanding scientific thoroughness "Penenomena of Materialization" by Baron Von Schrenck-Notzing who was a physician in Munich. This outstanding contribution to our knowledge of the hidden human personality was published by Kegan Paul in 1923.

The evidence witnessed by hundreds of medical and other men of science is as objective and convincing as photography and beyond the remotest suspicion of fraud. The research by all these outstanding people clearly shows that a discarnate intelligence has the power to produce certain astonishing and wonderful phenomena with the body of a physical medium of the calibre of Eva C. Eusapia Palladino, Rudi Schneider, Stanislava P. and many others.

From the plane or frequency rate of life's spectrum from which these discarnate intellects operate, they express a rate of vibration which is capable of disintegrating, or one could almost say dislodging ectoplasmic energy so as to extrude it from some orifices of the medium's body in varying degrees from cloud-like mist to threads and amorphous masses. The evidence shows that the medium cannot by her or his own will and desire produce these phenomena nor model in plastic form and in relief the hands, faces, bodies which were produced while these mediums were deeply entranced and not capable of functioning in a conscious mind.

This factual evidence obtained under conditions fulfilling all the requirements of scientific honesty, hence shows that a spirit or discarnate intelligence has the ability, or could attain it no doubt by a process of learning on the other side, to acquire the technique to produce ectoplasm such as have been indisputably observed.

The discarnate mind apparently employs some frequency rate of energy vibration which tunes in to the biological energy system of the medium, and so gradually intensifies or maybe increases the electric potential of a waveband of energy which in the examples provided by these physical mediums, is easily dislodged from its interassociations with other wavebands of the person's physiology.

If therefore a discarnate intelligence trained in the use of this power by means of thought, is capable of dislodging and extruding ectoplasm and moulding it into tangible objects, and then again allowing it to disintegrate and vanish into nothing before physical sight, can it equally not have the power to dematerialise a physical disease process by the concentration of ectoplasm in that area?

The possibility of such a process happening does not in the least seem absurd, but the actual occurrence of such a healing change would of course be dependent on the supply of ectoplasmic energy available within the body, and physiological functions of the sick person. The fact that only certain people are capable of supplying demonstrable ectoplasm and that these people are few and far between, indicates that if this theory of mine is the process by means of which faith or spiritual healing takes place, then the healing is conditioned by the strength of this waveband of energy available within the patient's body.

The healing of a wound where the protoplasmic strands resembling ectoplasmic threads ultimately become solid cells and fibrous tissue, has always been to me one of the deeper wonders of nature. From the day that the reality of the existence of the waveband of ectoplasmic energy could not any longer be excluded from my mind (if I were to be whole in my thinking of life) I saw this mysterious medium as the cohesive power of the organism; indeed a link between one's physical being and the insight and intelligence of the discarnate.

In reading these publications of ectoplasmic phenomena, and the productions of forms and photographs of those who have died, one is really astonished at the fact that the work of such men as Baron Von Schrenck-Notzing and Dr. Glen Hamilton have been allowed to fade into oblivion in an era when the intellect of man claims a disinterested curiosity as his scientific motivation. Will mankind not gain more by ascertaining the proper role of ectoplasm in our lives than spending millions on space prestige?

Those of us who believe that we have as scientific knowledge a selected perspective of the total man, can only draw attention to these frailties of the materialistic intellect, which makes science synonymous with knowledge, and in its limited vision denies our eternal spiritual values because its astronauts have not met spirits or God beyond our atmosphere and gravitational pull. Perhaps such statements by responsible men show that our inward vision is still nascent or degenerate.

In the work by Dr. Baron Von Schrenck-Notzing, Dr. Gustave Geley who was a psychologist and physician made certain interesting observations from which I would quote some of his impressions. Dr. Geley was like his colleague a scientific investigator and studied closely and lucidly the phenomena produced by the famous medium Eva C.

He described in detail how the substance emanated from the body of the medium, and then externalised itself in a sort of formless mass. Usually it first appeared as fluid, white and luminous flakes ranging from the size of a pea to that of a five-franc piece. The substance was seen distributed here and there over the medium's black dress, but principally on the left side of her body. The substance usually came from the mouth, the palate, nostrils, ears, eyes and from the mucous membrane of her cheeks, that is the inner surface, and also from her breasts around the nipples and from the top of her head on some occasions.

One is naturally interested to know what this substance is like to handle because of its property of becoming solid and then rapidly vanishing, not leaving a trace of physical existence. According to Dr. Geley's experience it occurred in various forms, sometimes displaying the property of being drawn out into a long thin thread or as he called it "ductile". There was an appearance and feeling resembling dough and at other times just a protoplasmic mass, that is a viscid, semi-fluid appearance, like the contents of our body cells.

The power of change or variation of appearance was of quite an extensive range, because the ectoplasm often appeared as numerous very thin threads, which apparently came together to form definite cords of varying thicknesses. Then all this would change and appear as narrow rigid rays or maybe some sort of self-luminous strands or rays of ectoplasm. Often it was seen as a broad band or as a fabric even as if it were some woven material. It actually at times assumed the appearance of a net or a large membrane with fringes and rucks.

Another interesting factor observed by these very able investigators was the behaviour of this substance. At times there was so much of it that it completely enveloped the medium, almost like a mantle. There was also a difference in colour, like the thin black cord which rang the bell in Dr. Glen Hamilton's experiments. The three colours carefully observed in the experiments with Eva C. were white, black and grey. The white was the most common, but at times it was seen that the visibility varied and slowly increased or decreased in succession.

It is tempting to draw certain conclusions from this change in colour of the ectoplasm. The thin black cord which came from a white mass and rang the electric bell for Dr. Hamilton could be the colour having a frequency for invisible movement of objects known as psychokinesis or in this case telekinesis. Perhaps the black ectoplasm is more resistant to light and might be a materialization in a field of force producing the peculiar poltergeist phenomena.

Dr. Geley described the sensation of touching the ectoplasmic substance as of a varying nature. Sometimes it was moist and cold like touching some reptile, I would say a snake or a worm. Then again the ectoplasm would be viscous and sticky, but more rarely it was actually dry and hard to the touch. The impression which this sensation gave to the mind depended on the shape which the substance assumed.

Many times the sensation was like feeling a spider's web with thin delicate strands sort of clinging around one's hand or face. Those who have walked into a big spider's web between two trees will accurately picture this variation of the ectoplasm. When however it was expanded into a large area like a mantle round the medium then it was delicately soft and elastic, but when it had to serve as a cord then it became knotty and fibrous like a piece of rope.

The observation of delicate threads like the strands of a spider's web gives the impression that the ectoplasm primarily and fundamentally appeared in this radiative thread form, and probably this condition at times gave the impression of rigid rays, but the threads were found to be both rigid and elastic. The mobility of the substance constituted another facet of interest. Its movements were those of a living substance and gravity had no effect on it.

The ectoplasmic manifestations consisted of movements slowly up and down across the medium's body, her shoulders, face and head in a sort of creepy motion, and it would curl over her breasts and right down to her knees. But this slow creepy, one could almost say exploring motion could change rapidly and become sudden and quick. It could also disappear like lightning and was shown again and again to have been extraordinarily sensitive. Now according to Dr. Geley this sensitivity of the ectoplasm was associated with the hypersensitivity of the medium herself.

I consider that this was an extremely interesting observation from a medical point of view. Patients who are extremely hypersensitive and so lay themselves open to being classed as neurotic and hysterical could be people whose ectoplasmic energy waveband of life's spectrum is more intensified than usual or than that of the average person. The human constitution still harbours many many secrets. It was found for instance with Eva C. that whenever the ectoplasmic extrusion was touched by someone the medium gave a painful reaction. Actually when the ectoplasmic substance was touched only moderately, but the touch was prolonged the medium complained and moaned that the pain was similar to an electric shock experienced by a normal body.

I think one could accept that this type of reaction of the medium shows that ectoplasm belongs to an inner aspect of the human personality. The fact that it seems to come primarily from orifices, the mucous membranes like those of the nose, eyes and mouth suggests its subtle role in the protoplasmic constituents of the human organism.

I have often wondered whether these predilections of the ectoplasm were not somehow related with certain functions of the astral body. Within the physical body could be these vortices of nervous energy forming generating centres in the astral, and so the ectoplasmic appearance becomes energy materialized by means of the operation of these centres corresponding to eyes, ears, nose, mouth and breasts in the outer physical being.

All observers have noticed the extreme sensitivity of this substance to ordinary light waves. Dr. Von Schrenck-Notzing in 1912 and onwards had to use magnesium flash for his photographs and he found that the medium reacted with a painful disturbance to sudden strong and unexpected light. Yet strangely enough this ectoplasmic substance in some cases was manifested as phenomena in full daylight. Hence we can speculate that it varies in its frequency rate of vibration and could at a certain rate be resistant to light waves. I consider that since ectoplasm was used as a medium for moving objects, and doing other invisible things it could at a certain rate of vibration be part of poltergeist phenomena.

Another characteristic of ectoplasm was its intrinsic, and as Dr. Geley called it irresistible tendency towards organization. It has its primitive or primary appearance which was observed if its rate of becoming something definite or growing into some object were not too rapid. It was almost as if at times it would produce its stages of becoming organized in slow motion so that the observer could follow its course from say cobweb threads to solid masses, cords and other resemblances to human organs.

But on other occasions the stages would follow with such rapidity that the human eye missed the sequence and the primary phases appeared not to have manifested at all. For example a soft elastic doughy mass would extrude itself from some of the source areas of the body, then a face would appear embedded in the amorphous ectoplasmic mass. The face could be like a flat photograph or it could be modelled and show characteristics of relief. So heads, faces and hands would appear. For example a mass of ectoplasmic substance would produce a finger from its fringe and then suddenly make it disappear.

The wonder of it all was the fact that the artists behind the scenes utilised the ectoplasmic substance to model various forms, and were able to impress by thoughtform photographs of discarnate beings, showing their identities with photographs then in existence. Once the modeller had produced and organized an organ he usually gave it a perfect appearance possessing all the biological qualities of a living organ. Fingers for example were produced from a mass of ectoplasm which were perfectly formed with beautiful life-like distinct nails.

The modelling of hands showed bones and joints. Dr. Geley wrote :

"I have seen a living head and felt the skull under thick hair, I have seen well-formed and living faces—human faces. In many instances these representations have grown under my own eyes from the beginning to the end of the phenomena."—"A head suddenly appears about thirty inches from the head of the medium above her and to the right side. It is a human head of normal dimensions well developed with usual relief. The top of the forehead and skull are completely materialised. The forehead is broad and high. The hair is short and thick and of a chestnut-brown colour."

These materialisations implied one or more discarnate intelligences moulding the ectoplasm into simulacra or likenesses of human organs. But the observations disclosed that these materialisations showed vitality in a biological sense. Actual faces appeared of people long dead, at first they were flat like pictures on paper and then grew into width, depth and length. These well-formed hands and faces were seen to dissolve into an ectoplasmic mass and then were reabsorbed into the body of the medium.

One of the most amazing materialisations was that of the little girl Rosalie as described by Harry Price in his book "Fifty Years of Psychical Research." The story of which I shall mention only brief excerpts begins with a Madame Z. whose husband was killed in 1916. She had a little daughter Rosalie who died of diphtheria at the age of six years. During 1925 Madame Z. was awakened during the night by the sound of her dead girl's voice crying "Mother".

This occurred so frequently that she used to lie awake at night listening for the voice. Gradually she thought she could see her in the dark and could hear little footsteps, while one night her hand was clasped by the little girl. Towards the end of 1928 regular seances were begun to encourage the visits of Rosalie. In 1929 Rosalie suddenly materialised and in complete darkness made her presence known by clasping her mother's hand.

Harry Price described how he visited the seance and what precautions he took against fraud, as he was determined to expose all mediums who aroused the slightest suspicion that fraudulent means might be employed to produce the effects. He made a tour of the house. "I had brought with me a gimlet, screw-eyes, white tape, adhesive surgical tape, a dredger full of powdered starch and a pocket torch (which I did not take into the seance room)."

He examined the house, closed and fastened each window and stuck a piece of tape across the join where the sashes met. He sealed all external doors and the French window with screw-eyes through which he threaded adhesive tape tied in three knots and which he then initialled. He was indeed nothing if not thorough.

In the seance room he stuck four strips of adhesive tape across the door and lintel and initialled them and treated the windows in the same manner. He was sure no one could enter that room, and even went so far as to place an evening newspaper on the top bar of the grate just under the chimney aperture in case anyone should come into the room that way. He sprinkled this thickly with starch and drew a monogram in the starch. No one could have tampered with the grate or chimney without disturbing the starch.

He examined everything in the room and each drawer of the sideboard was emptied. The settee was turned upside down, and he removed four rugs and opened the back of the wireless cabinet but could find nothing unusual. He was given permission to examine everyone present and he examined the men's clothing and contents. He sat between two spinster ladies whom he could not very well examine.

His last act before he turned out the lights was to sprinkle starch dust in front of the door and chimney after having directed all the sitters to their seats. "Four luminous plaques, hand mirrors covered with luminous paint, rested on the floor, face downwards, by the sides of the chairs occupied by Madame Z., Mrs. X., Jim and myself. The luminous surface of each plaque had been activated at an electric light bulb previous to the seance."

He then having taken every possible precaution against fraud described how he heard Madame Z. whisper the name "Rosalie" and he could hear Madame Z. and Mrs. X. sobbing quietly. Then later he described sensing something quite close to him and smelling a pleasant smell that was not previously there. He had the impression that the mother was fondling her child, and then he felt a slight touch on the back of his hand. His hand was resting on his knee and the touch on it was soft and a little warm. He sat quite still and made no attempt to feel what had touched him.

Then Mrs. X. asked Rosalie's mother whether Harry Price could touch the materialised form of the little girl. Now let Harry Price the famous exposer of mediums speak for himself.

"I stretched out my left arm, and, to my amazement it came in contact with, apparently, the nude figure of a little girl, aged six years.

"I slowly passed my hand across her chest up to her chin and cheeks. Her flesh felt warm, though (and this may have been my imagination) not so warm as one would expect to find normal human flesh. I laid the back of my left hand on her right cheek, it felt soft and warm, and I could distinctly hear her breathing. I then placed my hand again on her chest, and could feel the respiratory movement.

"I asked whether I could hold Rosalie. I was told that I could move my chair nearer to the child and this I did. I was now able to use both hands and again felt every inch of that little form. If it is a spirit—I argued to myself—then there is no difference between a spirit and a human being. With my right hand I lifted Rosalie's right arm and felt her pulse. I put my ear to her chest and could distinctly hear her heart beating.

"At this juncture I asked my hostess if Madame Z. would allow me to use the luminous plaque. I picked up my plaque and turning it over a soft fluorescent glow flooded the feet of Rosalie. They were the normal feet of a normal child. Mrs. X held the plaque to the left side of the girl while I illuminated the front of her. I could see the soft texture of the flesh which appeared without a blemish.

"As our plaques travelled upwards, the face was revealed and we beheld a beautiful child, who would have graced any nursery in the land. Her eyes (they appeared to be dark blue) were bright with an intelligent gleam in them. Madame Z said the examination must now cease as Rosalie was wanted. I was given one minute more to ask questions. 'Where do you live Rosalie?'—no answer. 'What do you do there?'—no answer. 'Do you play with other children?'—no answer. 'Have you any toys there?'—no answer. 'Are there any animal pets?'—no answer and then finally, 'Rosalie do you love your Mummy?' I saw the expression on her face change and her eyes light up. 'Yes' she whispered!"

The story of ectoplasm and materialisations have disclosed facts, inclusive of truths from reliable trustworthy sources. No rational approach imbued with the demand of scientific principle can fail to accept the evidence of the men I have mentioned as genuine in every sense of the word. Professor Richet, a famed physiologist was the first to recognize ectoplasm as a biological material. "*Thirty Years of Phychic Research*" by Charles Richet should be read by everyone who practises the profession of medicine.

There can be no argument, no dispute about the reality of the existence of ectoplasm, nor about the historical authentic recorded facts of the mediums who extruded this substance from their bodies. Dr. Von Schrenck-Notzing, with his well-known German thoroughness collected pieces of ectoplasm and handed these over to a chemical laboratory for expert examination and report.

The final analyses of the so-called ectoplasmic remains were found to contain the following :—

1. Large quantities of cell detritus and cell nuclei.
2. Large clear and well isolated plate epithelium cells in conjunction with various microbes.
3. Mucous-like substance with cell detritus and numerous microbes.
4. Some wool threads from the medium's dress.

The final result was that the ectoplasm as such had vanished leaving only remains of the cells of the body organ from which it was extruded. Hence ectoplasm can be accepted as a substance of organic origin and a component of man's body.

The experiments by the scientific-minded investigators who excluded the possibility of fraud by means of the techniques and procedures they employed showed that intelligences other than that of the entranced mediums controlled the phenomena. It appeared therefore that discarnate beings could exercise their artistic talents, and also their skills learned on the astral plane in the manipulation of the ectoplasmic substance which they by a process unknown to us disintegrated from the medium's cellular protoplasm and extruded through certain of her body orifices.

They utilised this material in the manner that a sculptor would do. They made hands, fingers, faces and whole bodies. Of course they were modelling with a living substance, and they were undoubtedly controlling the process of their creations by means of thought. Who knows but that this is a general law of life after death, whereby one has to learn to understand the hidden forces operating during physical life as though the inquiry of science is part of an eternal intellect.

When therefore a physical medium is available and trained for this purpose, it seems that discarnate entities work at the production of ectoplasm not only for our edification, but as a demonstration perhaps to other spirits who have to learn about life in all its manifestations.

They therefore indulge in the production of all sorts of images and objects and even material resembling woven cloth. Ectoplasm seems therefore to serve the creative impulse over there in the next world in the same manner as the potter's clay over here. But ectoplasm as part of the biological spectrum of organic substance must therefore occupy an inner degree of existence in the protoplasmic matter and energy of our body cells.

It does seem that in the case of little Rosalie her little astral body was covered by the ectoplasmic material available in the seance room. She was clothed in a substantial body tangible to touch with all the characteristics of life, because ectoplasm is one of the media of life. Therefore as a vehicle of life and an inner material of blood vessels, body cells, bones, hair, heart, brain and nerves even to the texture of the skin it could be extracted from people to make a biological garment for the astral body of little Rosalie.

But did the spirit of Rosalie so clothed in the vestment of a lower frequency energy system know how to utilise the ectoplasmic mechanism of direct voice? Surely these performances are not automatic but like all the higher laws of life as we know them demand a learning process? Little Rosalie appeared quite dumb to Harry Price's questions but was the ectoplasmic materialisation not a hindrance to her use of articulated speech? She might even have been confused by the new vehicle of her being. Her appearance was apparently to gratify her love for her mother and the mother's yearning for her. She was not concerned with other ideas except "Yes, I love Mummy."

We are of course also ignoring the possibility that a discarnate being who descends into energy systems of a lower order especially materialisation in ectoplasmic form, might suffer from an amnesia or a loss of memory for the higher planes of consciousness, and therefore little Rosalie could not find the right answers to Mr. Price's questions. It could be that materialisation of an astral form produces a strange state of consciousness which becomes limited in its intellectual powers. Perhaps the higher psychic functions are inhibited if not sacrificed for the building-up of an ectoplasmic organized body.

It could be said that Rosalie's inability to respond to Mr. Harry Price's questions in a simple intelligent manner indicated that the form however life-like had no intelligent comprehension or spiritual intelligence. But when we refer to Dr. Glen Hamilton's experiments it is mentioned by the controlling spirit named Walter that in building up the ectoplasmic forms and objects he had not sufficient power or energy available also to produce the ectoplasmic mechanism for a direct voice communication.

Here then is evidence of some conservation of energy for a particular purpose and that purpose was to extrude and demonstrate ectoplasm as a peculiar form of matter quite unknown to science. This demonstration also showed that it was pliable to spirit thought control and that it could act as a photographic plate and reveal pictures in miniature form of those who lived on earth. The direct voice hence required that a special voice production mechanism had to be built by means of ectoplasm before direct voice speech could be heard.

Experience has revealed to many investigators in this branch of psychic research that the use of the direct voice as a form of communication by a discarnate was a process that had to be learned. The first attempts were usually poor in articulation and were frequently just a mumble. Evidently this mechanism had to be constructed out of ectoplasmic and astral components and thereafter the discarnate intellect had to learn the skill of certain forms of energy-control and rhythm to produce a spoken voice, recaptured as it were from earthly memories.

It is quite possible that in the case of little Rosalie the spirit controls were fully aware that Mr. Price acted as a psychic research sleuth with his nose to the ground looking for fraud. They therefore produced a phenomenon of a living being from a system of energy over which they had control and which vanished with the material form of Rosalie. This energy was drawn by these spirit-beings from the medium and those present including the physical organism of Mr. Price. It was a supreme effort for conviction of the continuation of life, for them to have modelled the biological form of Rosalie.

I am quite sure that according to the statements of the spirit control Walter in Dr. Glen Hamilton's series, that conservation of energy, and the process of making an ectoplasmic vocal mechanism, as well as the learning of the skill of how to use this mechanism, were all factors which prevented Rosalie from entering into a conversation with Mr. Price.

It should also be remembered that it was after Mr. Price was told that Rosalie had to leave that he asked the questions. This could imply that there was not only Rosalie's inability to employ intelligently the ectoplasmic vocal mechanism, but there was insufficient power left for such an effort, except to say "Yes" in a gentle soft voice to the question whether she loved her Mummy.

It is natural for us to assume that the direct voice requires a laryngeal mechanism with vocal cords such as we possess physically, but this mechanism in its ectoplasmic form may be quite different and operate on a level and range of vibrations which require learning and adaptation in the next world.

For the spirit controls to have produced this wonderful demonstration of organised substance from invisible sources of man, and so revealed to the most critical investigator a biological being with all its aesthetic qualities, was indeed an achievement with a profound purpose for man. Later on we shall speculate about this purpose in the life of the evolution of consciousness.

These manifestations support the spiritistic hypothesis, because no one in that room could by the power of their minds have produced and modelled this reproduction of a physical being. These things are beyond the powers of physical man, because I think it requires a special skill to employ this energy system of a spectrum of life, which we cannot acquire or learn to perform while in the physical state. Dr. Glen Hamilton for instance said :— "The introduction of an intelligence—some manner of intelligence—is imperative and necessary to any explanation of the phenomena. This by evidence is inescapable. This incompatibility can best be resolved in our opinion by the introduction of a theory of a discarnate or non-living intelligence."

The New Testament presents us with numerous psychic phenomena and it is apparent judging from this evidence that the disciples and others associated with Jesus were decidedly psychic. Jesus himself gives the impression of having been a great medium not only in psychic diagnosis but in many other respects. I have for instance often wondered whether his walking on the water was plain levitation or an astral projection?

The most interesting psychic manifestation came after his death. In St. John 20 verse 14 we read :— "And when she thus said, she turned herself back, and saw Jesus standing, and knew not that it was Jesus." This surely suggests that he was not in his usual physical form, and that she could have seen an astral vision of him clairvoyantly and did not recognize him in that form and presentation, which was probably self-luminous as has been observed in others even in our times.

Altogether he is said to have made ten appearances after his physical death. All these could be taken as demonstrations of the survival of the psyche, but the one that is of profound interest and which should in all respects be considered as a materialisation is where he presented proof of his identity to Thomas. I am prepared to accept the others as falling within the category of clairvoyant visions because many of his disciples could have had this astral vision.

The evening of his materialisation as presented in St. John 20 verses 26, 27 and 30 cannot be considered as in any way different from those manifestations which psychic research investigators have observed. The Bible states :— "And after eight days again his disciples were within and Thomas with them : then came Jesus, the doors being shut, and stood in the midst, and said Peace be unto you."

We observe that emphasis is laid on the doors being shut. Therefore the impression is conveyed that one must not think in terms of him having entered the room by normal means. In other words it was not a physical entrance of one with a material body.

He came to manifest from an invisible to a tangible and visible degree in their midst. The question that has often come to my mind when reading of this occasion is whether those disciples were not actually conducting a seance at that time?

In any case he materialised. "Then saith he to Thomas, Reach hither they finger, and behold My hands : and reach hither they hand, and thrust it into my side : and be not faithless without believing." Therefore this ectoplasmic form produced by him from the psychic powers of His disciples was of such a potential that he could produce his wounds and he could produce speech. The manifestation was so tangible that Thomas who could not imagine man's abstract form had to admit the reality of the objective ectoplasmic reproduction of the marks of the crucifixion.

In verse 30 it is written :— "And many other signs truly did Jesus in the presence of his disciples, which are not written in this book." These signs therefore must concern rites and symbols known to his disciples which he employed to establish his identity. How many of the thousands of men and women who have read this chapter in the Bible have ever associated this appearance of Jesus after his death with the well-known physical phenomena of materialisation?

When we think of the living and beautiful reproduction of Rosalie then this appearance of Jesus to his disciples and especially Thomas shows the same mechanism and the same substance as observed by the pioneers of psychic research including Mr. Harry Price. It is almost as though the same eternal truth with the same significance and connotation was demonstrated by little Rosalie with Mr. Price perhaps unwittingly playing the role of Thomas in the twentieth century.

CHAPTER IX

"SOUTH AFRICAN ASTRAL EXPERIENCES"

If we accept the existence of an astral body made of a substance constituting the inner personality of man, then life offers us a promise of adventure once we have left the biological requirements of the other physical personality. Without this conception of the astral vehicle of Ego and its consciousness, we are doomed to live in ignorance of our own inner splendour. Our own potentialities of achievement will remain hidden in the veiled depths of our magnificence. Life seems to have made it a natural task for man to accept himself through the crust of materialism with which he is enveloped.

It is highly possible that our emergent penetration through the denser layers of the human mind may eventually reveal to man a body of compact light; for already we live a creative life, and by means of that wonderful faculty of imagination, thought becomes a reality for the creation of many forms and patterns whose aesthetic appeal require a materialised appearance.

Mind has seen the light of day by means of its sense equipment. This tangible reality has been its first love in life, and all its instinctive needs were primarily gratified by physical means, where the resistance of matter made the real world. It is therefore very difficult and oft times incomprehensbile for the human mind to even allow itself to imagine a deeper reality than its physical form.

There seems almost an aggressive hopelessness in the tone of voice of the person who somehow feels a personal if not egotistic distinction in saying "I believe that when you are dead you are dead." But of course no one will dispute this shallowness of thought, which the person thinks is profound, as long as he confines himself to the outer vehicle of the Ego known as the body. If however he includes man's consciousness and power of thought as well, and accepts that these constitute a form of energy, and that energy is indestructible, then man's inner being as the source of thought is equally made of energy and thus indestructible.

If therefore we study the experiences of people, which provide evidence of this higher energy system of the astral being, our conclusions can in no way be considered less rational than those that accept the existence of the 'electron' as a disembodied charge of electricity. The human experience that has been placed at my disposal concerning this phenomenon of leaving the physical body during life for short periods will speak with its own sincerity and honesty.

Mrs. Greyling of Ohrigstad wrote to me in Afrikaans of an interesting separation of her astral self, during a period of unconsciousness. But before we come to this particular experience I would like to mention that Mrs. Greyling has had many other psychic experiences from an early age and her mother as well had a similar personality make-up. As a little girl Mrs. Greyling had premonitions of illness in her family and at times precognitive visions or actual visions of happenings concerning her loved ones that had taken place hundreds of miles away.

I am mentioning these associated phenomena of clairvoyance and precognition to show that the person capable of remembering and recalling the events of an astral separation from the physical body has undoubtedly a tendency to ready dissociation between the astral body and the physical outer vehicle of the psyche. This separation must be dependent on an unusual interassociation of the various energy systems which go to form the personality and its different degrees of consciousness.

Mrs. Greyling had a little sister who was quite well at the time, and yet one day she saw a vision of a little girl closely resembling her little sister who kept appearing to her and winking at her, smiling as if highly amused at something which Mrs. Greyling did not know or suspect. This vision frightened her and she did not want to stay by herself in the house during the day. She recognized that the vision was that of her baby sister and then three months later this child died.

She described her stay in a sanatorium while suffering from tuberculosis. She was there for eighteen months during which time she had an operation which was performed in two stages. It was during the second stage that something went wrong according to what she learned from the doctors and her husband after her recovery. They would not give her details but said she was almost dying. She was unconscious from the Tuesday when they operated until the Thursday when she regained physical consciousness.

My translation of her extraordinary experience is as follows :

"The first awareness that I remember was of standing in front of my bed and seeing thereon my physical body. I looked at it but felt really very little, if any, interest in it. I saw it covered with blankets and hot-water bottles. I then became conscious of my own new self. I felt wonderful. It is difficult to describe how sublimely wonderful I felt. My body had no weight, it was light and I did not stand on the earth, or the floor of the ward, but was suspended as if floating in my movements—an exhilarating buoyancy filled my being.

"What however was strange was that when I was near my body

I felt the heaviness and the pain in that physical body on the bed. Somehow my proximity to the physical body on the bed made me in some mysterious way feel its sensations in my new body, but as I moved away from it these sensations of heaviness and pain decreased until I reached a point in distance when I no longer felt them, although I was fully conscious that it was my body lying there on the bed, all covered up with blankets.

"I wish I could precisely describe in language the difference as I felt it between being in my new body and the awful distress and pain that was going on in my physical body, but really I have no adequate language for this experience. And yet I must tell you doctor that I was tremendously interested and keenly aware of this sort of dual consciousness of being elated and happy in my new body and miserable and in great pain in my physical body, but this only was felt when I came very near to my old body on the bed."

This very profoundly interesting description bears out Sylvan Muldoon's experience with regard to the range of the astral cable or cord. Mrs. Greyling went on :

"I stood for a while in front of my bed looking at my body and feeling all the sensations of the physical body when I approached too near, and then decided to move away from my old body with all its unpleasant feelings. I turned towards the door and was conscious of moving with such floating grace, that it was the most pleasant feeling I had ever lived; I could really say that I could ever have imagined.

"In this delightful mood of freedom and effortless movement, as if the power that moved me was just a mere desire or a thought, I found myself going down the long passage of the sanatorium and into the large ward which I shared with several other female patients before I went to the operating theatre. I stood next to their beds and passed from one to the other, after all we were friends and had been in that ward together for months. I smiled and spoke but no one saw or heard me. I realized that the form and life which I possessed was invisible to their eyes, neither could they hear my words.

"When I found that I made no impression on them, I turned and made for the door. But now something strange happened, I became aware of a male person whose body was of the same translucent substance as mine walking along with me on my right side. I looked at him but could not distinguish his face. The features were not clearly defined, they seemed to have been covered with some haziness.

"What was strange to me was the absence of nervousness, or fear or discomfort in the presence of this man who kept pace with me, and moved in the same gliding effortless manner by my side.

I remember having the thought that he somehow belonged to me, as if he were there silently to protect me. I felt marvellously contented, and seemed to understand deep inside me that this person was really some sort of a guardian or guide who came to meet me and introduce me to my new life.

"Without any curiosity or any emotion such as I would have had experience if this had happened in my physical life, I just took it all for granted, and so walked on in his company. At first we went uphill. I remember distinctly this incline and tendency to steepness as we walked on air, side by side along what I thought was a footpath. I am sure that the little footpath had green grass on either side.

"Now while we were ascending this incline, I became conscious of a voice calling my name. It was a man's voice, and I heard it distinctly. It kept on calling earnestly and almost, so to speak, in a pleading voice. I say this because I could register all the feelings in the voice as if in a flash. My new mind was ever so much keener, so that I could feel a thousand different thoughts and emotions in that voice which called 'Lola, Lola, come back Lola. Come back, don't don't go away yet. Please come back.' As I heard the voice I knew what it contained. I knew all its feelings and yet I was in such a serene and delightful frame of mind that only a part of me heard the call.

"Then it seemed to invade my consciousness and became more and more pressing, pleading and almost begging me to return. At this I for the first time became aware of concern. It began to worry me. It was just the same as if one were called away from some pleasant task to the most mudane and uninteresting duty. 'Lola come back' came like an echo through the heavens.

"The power of the voice began to move all my feelings. I turned to my silent companion and said I was sorry, very sorry, that I could not accompany him. I said : 'Do you hear how he is calling me. I must go back. You will understand that that voice needs me.' It seemed as if at that moment everything faded into nothing. The flow of memory just snapped and ceased, because I who remembered every detail from the time that I was out of my body had no memory from the moment I decided to return until I regained earthly consciousness on the Thursday.

"When I became aware of where I was on the third day after my operation I was packed around with hot-water bottles, and the nurse said that the doctors had expected me to die. I have never forgotten this vital memory, it is now eleven years ago. My husband and my two small children prayed and prayed for my return during those days when, according to the nurse, 'your life was hanging on the thinnest of threads.' "

A lady who wished to remain anonymous wrote in English about her experience out of the physical body. In spite of this extremely impressive and convincing event in her life she has been unable to accept the idea of survival after death.

She wrote :

"About twenty years ago when I was thirty-six I had an experience of astral projection but was not at all ill. I had had a major operation a few months previously but had recovered and was holding down a strenuous job. I went to sleep on a Saturday afternoon—a quite dreamless and untroubled sleep, when suddenly I became aware that I was up in the roof of my room, looking down at my sleeping body lying on the bed on the other side of the room. It was just a flash but it made an indelible impression on my mind—when I woke I felt far away for an hour or so.

Of course I never mentioned it to anyone, not wanting to be thought 'bats' and was most surprised when a few years back I discovered a book in a Durban library which explained astral projection. I still do not believe in a hereafter. I feel that just as our physical bodies disintegrate in the earth after death, probably the astral body, which is the real us does the same into thin air. I hope so anyway."

I do not deny that ultimately in the evolution of consciousness the astral will have to be discarded, so man in his transformation dies a second time. But my correspondent has confused the vehicle with the dynamic and activating consciousness, the generator of thought, whose integrity of continued existence finds its corollary in the law of conservation of energy.

Anyway my correspondent mentioned another experience which could quite easily have been an astral projection rather than a projection of a thoughtform. She went on :

"Then a few years ago I had a telepathic experience. I woke one night early from a peaceful sleep (in a room that was locked and burglar-proofed) to see my chief at the office standing beside my bed in the flesh it seemed. He was in evening dress with dinner jacket; he was gazing intently at me and with a most hostile expression on his face, and as I looked at him he vanished into thin air.

"This puzzled me (it was before I had read the book on psychic phenomena). I soon put it out of my mind, but the experience was explained a few months later when I made an unpleasant discovery and was forced to expose the poor man to head-office. He must have been very worried and distressed that night and was no doubt wondering what action I would take. Poor man, it was most tragic."

Let us assume that this gentleman had worried over his misappropriation of funds maybe, and that after dinner and a fair amount of alcohol (for she discovered that he was an alcoholic as well) he fell asleep in his evening clothes with the dominant idea in his mind that an exposure was bound to come. He knew of no way in which he could prevent her from revealing his fraud. Perhaps he thought of silencing her in some manner, with the result of an astral projection in an angry mood and in a form that appeared to her as one in the flesh.

Miss Sheila Wahl who had many psychic experiences described a phantom appearance of a surgeon while she was awake. Her account of this event when she suffered tremendous pain from a facial neuralgic condition had best be left to her own description.

"On the following Saturday I was lying wide awake on my face and in great pain, when I felt a tap on my left shoulder. I turned my head and saw this surgeon standing beside my bed. He said: 'You have nothing to worry about—your X-rays are absolutely normal.' So I said aloud 'Oh'—he replied 'No—don't look so disappointed—I'll cut the gland out if you want me to do so.' I smiled and said I had thought that at last they had found the cause of the pain in one side of my face. He thereupon disappeared.

"On the Monday following, I had to report at the hospital for the results of the X-rays and as I walked into the room the surgeon said: 'Your X-rays are absolutely normal—you have nothing to worry about.' Then he said: 'Don't look so disappointed—I'll cut the gland out if you want me to do so,' and I almost said 'You've told me that before.' "

I have since spoken to one of the doctors who attended to Miss Wahl and there was quite a discussion on the cause of her facial pain. The surgeon too was puzzled. It is therefore highly probable that on the Saturday night when Miss Wahl was in pain and at home this surgeon was thinking of her condition and had perhaps already seen the X-ray plates; he was therefore happy in his mind that the condition was not as serious as they thought. Then during his sleep his astral body under the impulse of his sympathy for the patient visited her, and said the exact words which he repeated on the Monday.

Miss Wahl once conversed regularly with what she thought was a spirit over a period of three years. But this spirit who so frequently appeared to her wore a beard. She must have seen him in quite an objective form. Then one day she met this so-called spirit-man actually in the flesh, and the first thing he said to her was: "Where have I seen you before?" Then he showed her a large photograph of himself with a beard, just as she had seen him on his visits, and before she could say anything he said "Yes I shaved my beard off three days ago."

This particular experience of Miss Wahl's is most interesting, because she being psychic saw this apparition, whom she thought was a spirit. They had long telepathic conversations when he visited her and he even gave her a name by which to call him. During these appearances she was awake and not therefore asleep or in a state of astral projection. But the so-called spirit could have been no other than this gentleman in astral form visiting a person for whom he had a great affinity.

The following letter in Afrikaans from which I quote the significant material is so plainly sincere and honest that it is worth its place among those who have experienced a journey into space in astral form. Mrs. G. of Lydenburg described her experience in this manner :

"Something most extraordinary happened to me in March 1961. I was ill and had a high temperature and my heart was giving trouble at the same time. I was in bed and felt deeply depressed.

"My thoughts were frightening—what would happen to my only little girl and my husband should I die? They needed me so much. I felt so ill that I really thought I would not live a few days longer. Anyway somehow I fell asleep. About three o'clock in the morning I woke and to my utter surprise I found myself gliding through our bedroom door. I was near the top of the door and at that moment looked back towards the bed and there was my exhausted body. It looked lifeless to me. I was about fifteen feet from where my husband was sleeping.

"I thought that this was the end of my physical existence, and that death had brought a change for a new life. But at that moment I thought of my little daughter and how she would miss me. As these ideas about her went through my mind I suddenly felt a strange uncomfortable repercussive effect and there was I wide awake and back in my sick and painful body."

Mr. Badenhorst of Lichtenburg wrote to me about an experience which he considered to have been a separation of his spirit from his body. I shall adhere as closely as possible to his excellent descriptive Afrikaans version of this event.

"I was lying on my back and snoring aloud. This is a family habit, we all snore terribly. Then I became aware in that dream-state that a nebulous sparkling golden substance, but which was not matter or material in a physical sense, was streaming or radiating out of my body.

"There was my body which in my dream was motionless, but this strange translucent golden greyish cloud-form became a sort of covering, a configuration within which was my body. And then it moved away from my body—it stretched leaving a band attached to my body but this became thinner and thinner. Yet the farther this phantom moved from my body the brighter and more brilliant it became.

"But along the cord which still attached this phantom-being of golden white light to my body, there sparkled like a million diamonds tiny dancing spots of brilliance. I immediately wanted to resist this separation of body and soul. I was actually afraid to give up my earthly existence for the uncertainty of the unknown world to which I feared I was drifting. Then somehow this fearful emotion was counteracted by a strange happiness, a feeling of freedom and delightful detachment which flowed together into anticipation of that future.

"I was aware that I rested on the boundary line, an unnamed frontier between two media of existence. Here was the line of crossing from grey-darkness to light—supreme living light, and from evil in our world to serene kindness and goodness. At that moment I knew a new reality, timeless yet positive as though it made me realize the glory of one's inner self. I felt my earthly passions melting away and I could understand their uses to the physical body.

"I woke on terra firma and I thought and wondered a great deal about this amazing dream-picture. I came to the conclusion that death was not what we feared and that it has many correspondencies with birth." Mr. Badenhorst does not tell us where he thought the seat of his consciousness was during this dream-experience of other-worldly mystic grandeur. And yet I think that this was an experience of his astral consciousness because he became aware of a distinction between his new or inner feeling-state at home in a higher self and the passions, instincts and needs of his physical being.

Here are a few more experiences of the psychic sensitive Miss Sheila Wahl. "Some years ago I had a conscious passing into spirit! I was aware of the fact that I was leaving my body, through the chest, and then I stood beside my bed and surveyed my body, but I was not really interested in it. I then floated to the ceiling and felt it touching my back and I wanted to 'go.'

I looked at the silver ribbon, about two inches wide connecting me with my body, and I surveyed the room and its contents, my sister asleep and the dogs, and then I saw Stanley the soldier friend who had died in Italy on 7th February 1945. He was tugging at my skirt, so to speak, and saying 'No you can't go now, you must come back.' I said 'Come on Stanley, let's go,' and all I wanted to do was to float out of the fanlight above the door.

He tugged at me hard and said 'No—not now' with alarm in

his voice. Then I realized that I was coming back into my body and I tried desperately to get out again, but I only managed half-way and then I was back in my body. I had pins and needles in my feet and a feeling of great disappointment assailed me."

In this astral projection which Miss Wahl called "passing into spirit" she was completely conscious during the whole process except for a brief gap as the complete interassociation between the astral and the physical took place, and then to regain consciousness knowing all that had transpired. What is of interest was the meeting with Stanley. Miss Wahl did not say whether she was thinking of him at the time and whether there was some longing to meet him again.

The evidence of many people strongly suggests that astral travel is quite common except that few people retain a clear memory of the experience. I should say that in most people the return to integration with the physical body produces an amnesia, which goes back in time and so covers the period when out of the body.

It probably has a vague resemblance as regards memory loss to a severe contusion to the brain, or a commotion of the brain as a result of injury, commonly motor accidents when the memory is lost for events preceding the impact up to half-an-hour sometimes. The return of the astral always seems to break the continuity of consciousness, which suggests the organic role of ectoplasm re-establishing its previous electro-magnetic contacts. Memory is probably lost when this contact is formed on re-integration.

Miss Wahl related another experience of an astral visit from a friend. "During the war I was expecting a soldier friend to visit me from camp, but something intervened and he was not able to come. I went to bed early and although my room was semi-light from the reflection of a light from the passage the rest of the house was lit up. I was awake when all of a sudden I felt as if bees were buzzing in my ears and I got pins and needles in my feet.

Then I beheld this soldier in uniform standing in the middle of the room. He appeared to be pushing people aside as if to get nearer to me. He then appeared right next to my bed and sat down on it and I felt the bed go down with his weight. He then lay down next to me on his right elbow and I was conscious of the red tab on his left shoulder and I felt the weight on the bed and the pillow. The buzzing and pins and needles dwindled and the vision faded. I then called my brother and told him about it. Was it a thought-form?"

There were certain physical sensations associated with this apparition of a soldier who was alive at the time. Miss Wahl felt pins and needles and her ears were buzzing. These manifestations indicated that a change was taking place in her metabolism and that some bio-electric disturbance was present. In other words power was being drawn from her mediumistic body.

We do not know whether at that time this soldier was asleep in camp or whether he was experiencing a conscious astral projection by imagining himself in her company and wishing it. In any case the materialisation became so solid with its dense ectoplasmic covering that she felt the sensation of weight on her bed. A mere thoughtform could hardly produce these life-like tangibilities, but then there is the possibility that Miss Wahl provided the power for his materialisation. I have since wondered whether this was Stanley who called her back to her body. Miss Wahl was apparently aware that the soldier who came to life on her bed was not of flesh and blood.

Mrs. K. who wished to remain anonymous wrote in Afrikaans from Pretoria. "I want to tell you about my experience as briefly as possible and I would very much prefer not to have my name mentioned for reasons which you will understand. But please do not doubt the truth of my letter. I was a mother of five children and lost one of them a few years ago. I was very tired and exhausted from deep depression, worry and hard work. I felt completely without energy and decided to lie down on my bed and rest a while at about two o'clock in the afternoon.

"Now I do not remember for how long I was lying on my bed. I had lost my son of nineteen in April 1958 as a result of a motor car accident. He was in the army and a few of them were killed at Muldersdrift. Well his death made me so sorrowful and depressed that there were times when I lived as an automaton. Then I began to comtemplate suicide, and felt convinced that I could not continue in that frame of mind, and that death by my own hand was the only way out. That afternoon when I went to lie down to think of suicide, it was just four months since his death.

"Then as from nowhere my soldier son appeared and stood before my bed. He was in uniform and I could see his corporal's stripes. He was brown from the sun the way he always looked in life. Then with some effort he spoke and said : 'Mother see for yourself I am alive—I am living. I am not dead the way you think' and with that he vanished into nothing.

"He was killed on the 19th of April 1958 and ever since on the date of his death he has appeared to me. Sometimes without his tunic and his cap, and at other times in full uniform, and always he has had something encouraging to say to me, and to impress on my mind that he existed and was alive and found his new life tremendously interesting. From his first appearance in that solid body so vital and real I have become a different person and have realized that he came to rescue me from what I contemplated.

I must tell you what happened after his first appearance. I was again lying down in the afternoon when it seemed as if I went into a slumber, and at once I found myself up near the ceiling of my room. There was my body lying on the bed and here was I somewhere in the air.

I then began to hover and came down to about three feet above my body on the bed. Then I moved away again and closely observed every article of furniture and other knickknacks in the room. I went outside, so lovely and free and peaceful, and saw my little daughter of three playing with her toys, and my husband hard at work in an outbuilding.

Please understand me, this was no dream because all that happened where my husband was working and what he was doing I saw in my new body outside the house while my physical body was on the bed. I could see what they were doing but they could not see me, and yet I knew this was the same sort of new body which my son had, for I felt life as something so different, as if the most glorious feelings were flowing to this new body from some profound far-away source. It was too wonderful."

This letter in its simple Afrikaans is pregnant with plain honesty. The fact that Mrs. K. experienced an astral projection showed that she was unconsciously mediumistic and in all probability provided the power by means of which her son could materialise his astral form.

A Mr. de K. a student of Pretoria University communicated with me in Afrikaans about his own experience and those of a friend in attempting voluntary astral projection by means of concentration. His friend became somewhat frightened after his first awareness of being out of his physical body, and thereafter gave it up for a time because when he found himself out of his physical body he thought he was dead and this terrified him. I suppose he had a sort of repercussive effect.

After he had overcome his early anxieties he tried again and succeeded in existing in his astral form completely away from his body. He also found that he often visited a little village in his astral body, which a friend of his who also projected astrally described to him as one of the familiar scenes of his journeys on the astral plane. His friend made several interesting observations while in the astral form. He found for example that he could differentiate a multitude of wonderful colours in that atmosphere. These were aesthetically supremely impressive.

According to Mr. de K.'s letter there are several students at Pretoria and Stellenbosch Universities who are experimenting with astral projection. I am sure that the Society for Psychic

Research of the Witwatersrand University would be extremely grateful to receive data of these most laudable psychic research projects by intelligent young men of our universities.

A charming letter from East London under the *nom de plume* of Astra (although the real name is known to me) describes an experience which cannot be anything else but astral projection during an illness guided by the affinities of friendship and sympathy. She wrote : "Three weeks ago I was very ill with pneumonia and was delirious one night, during which time my best friend who lives in England (Suffolk) saw me in her bedroom and she had not yet gone to bed.

The strange part about it was that she saw me as I used to be years ago and also as I am now after a recent operation for cancer. She sat down immediately and wrote to me and I received this letter a few days later, when it crossed my note to her telling her of my sudden and almost fatal illness."

My correspondent "Astra" is also a clairvoyant and has had premonitory and precognitive experiences. Her constitution therefore belongs to the mediumistic or psychic sensitive class in whom I think the magnetic interassociations and integrations of the various energy systems holding the astral in the physical are not so firmly adherent or adhesive as in most of us. Hence during her serious illness her astral body loosened itself and went to her friend and most intelligently conveyed the significance of change due to illness by giving two pictures, the one before and the one after an operation for cancer. Did the astral intellect do this by itself or was it assisted, as Dr. Glen Hamilton's work has shown?

Mrs. Hunter, Junior Red Cross organizer for the Eastern Cape told me of an interesting astral experience as a child. She was in a terrible train smash in the Cape and suddenly came to herself quite free and alive but to her amazement saw her twisted, badly cut and bleeding unconscious body in the wreckage. She remembers saying to herself : "Oh my here am I killed in this train smash and now I shall never be able to fulfill my ambition to write a novel." She saw the rescuers at work while she floated as it were in her ethereal body and then suddenly it happened, she regained consciousness in her body torn with pain.

Mr. Sadie who so kindly placed his manuscript in Afrikaans at my disposal records an interesting case of astral projection by Sister G. Heinz a masseuse at the warmbaths near Carolina. He knew her well and therefore this account of her experiences is of special interest. She told him how profoundly astonished she was when for the first time she found herself outside her body.

At that time she was living in a flat in Eloff Street in Johannesburg. One afternoon she decided to lie down and rest a while on her bed. What happened after lying down she could not remember but came to herself floating out of a third-floor window of the block of flats and on her back in the position which she occupied on the bed. When she realized where she was and in what state she was gripped by terror and immediately found herself in her body with terrific repercussion and with her heart racing at a great speed.

A few days later she told a friend in Kensington about her unusual experience of floating in the air. The friend then assured her that it was a harmless and interesting experience and invited her to come and visit them in her astral body on the next occasion on which she found herself in a similar state.

Some days later she woke from a sound sleep and found herself standing next to her bed looking at her own body lying on the bed asleep. She immediately thought of her friend's invitation and as it was still early in the evening she decided to go visiting. She turned round to leave the room and it appeared to her as if she actually opened the door. Then standing in front of the lift she realized that she would not be able to press the button, and so decided to walk down the stairs.

Once in the street she wondered whether to take the tram but decided that as she had no money, she would walk along the tram-lines to Kensington. Next she found herself in front of the garden gate of the house where her friend stayed, and here she faced a problem—they would not be able to see her she thought, and therefore the visit appeared to her somewhat absurd. In the end she decided to return to her flat but could not remember how she reached her room except that she woke in bed with a clear memory of her journey and her impressions.

The next day she decided to go to Kensington and visit her friend in the flesh. To her amazement her friend greeted her with the words : "Why did you not come in last night? I saw you at the gate." Sister Heinz then told her friend about her experience and how she had walked along the tram-lines from Eloff Street to Kensington. Her friend was greatly amused and told her not to think in terms of walking but all she had to do the moment she found herself in her astral body was to think of her destination and form a clear picture in her mind of the place she wants to visit, thereafter she would probably find her intentions fulfilled.

After this conversation with her friend weeks passed without any feeling of astral projection or any consciousness of a disturbance of that nature. Then one evening whilst lying on her bed she came to herself some distance from the bed and there and then made up her mind to form a clear picture of her friend's house. At once she felt herself moving through space and within a short time was outside the little gate of the house.

Once there she was puzzled what to do and felt that she could not just enter the house without knocking or in some way announcing her presence. She decided to knock in the hope that the people of the house would hear the knock on the door. What was her surprise when she heard footsteps within coming towards the door and there stood the lady of the house with whom her friend boarded; but what was more bewildering to her was that the lady said : "Oh Sister Heinz I am so glad that you could come."

The lady then told her that her little boy was sick and so she accompanied her to the bedroom to the sick child. From this moment her memory became vague but she remembered trying to arrange the blankets on the child's bed and the next moment she was back in bed in her own flat. Some days later she actually visited her friend in the flesh and as she came in the lady of the house said : "Wherever did you go to the other night? I only left the room for a moment to fetch something for my little boy and when I returned you had gone." It is apparent that Sister Heinz must have been seen in a very dense astral form or perhaps the lady was clairvoyant? Anyway she thought that she had seen Sister Heinz in her physical body. Mr. Sadie had no more to say about whether Sister Heinz continued to experiment with her astral projections or not. An interesting feature of her experiences however was the habitual functions of the mind especially the way she made her astral body walk as if it were physical because she did not know the power of wish on the astral self. On the second occasion she merely pictured her goal and then felt the movement very much in the manner described by my typhoid patient.

Mr. Sadie mentions the experience of Mr. H. J. van Staden of Pretorius Street, Wesselsbron. He described how he was lying on his back on his bed with his hands under his head. He was wide awake and he was contemplating getting up. It was fairly early in the morning and the sun had not yet risen. Lying there thinking of the day and its work and all its other implications he became aware of the presence of a strange girl in the house.

From his bed his vision included a portion of the lounge as the door was open. He could see the farthest wall of the lounge against which hung a huge oil painting. The girl was standing facing the picture with her back towards him and whilst looking at the painting she brushed her hair, or stroked it, backwards with both her hands, and her attitude was that of someone looking at the picture as though it were a huge mirror.

While lying there speechless with wonder and marvelling at the display revealed by his vision, she turned round and faced him, and once more stroked her hair with a graceful backward movement. Then she smiled sweetly at him as if to say "that it is no longer time for sleep." He saw her so plainly and distinctly that he could see her features and facial expression as well as her clothes.

He saw that she had bright blue eyes with a lovely skin, pure milk-white and very smooth. Her nose was sharp and somewhat pointed but did not detract from the rest of her beautiful face. Her dress was rose-coloured and of a floral design with a silky appearance. After she had stood and looked at him for a few moments, while he was lying there tongue-tied with amazement, she turned again to face the picture, and he noticed that she had lovely long blonde hair which reached down well below her shoulders. Again her hand came over stroking her hair as if she enjoyed the feel of its solftness and texture. One could almost say she was admiringly caressing her hair. Then she turned sideways and looked at him with the same sweet mischievous smile. After that she somehow just stepped aside and vanished.

Later that day he told the other members of his family about this strange and beautiful phantom visitor. Then to his surprise he discovered that his father had also seen her and could describe her features, expression and general appearance in the same detail as he had observed them. They had no idea who she could have been and where she could have come from. They never saw her again in their home, but a year later his father was at some social gathering and there to his utter astonishment was the same girl in the flesh; yes the identical personality. One regrets that neither Mr. van Staden nor his father followed up this interesting case of evident astral projection.

Mr. Sadie also described a vision seen by Mrs. Jack Nel of Nelspruit. She said : "I woke one night to find that my husband was standing in the bedroom dressed in his pyjamas. I turned my head to look next to me and there was his physical body fast asleep. I was so bewildered at this strange spectacle that I did not know what to do. I could not understand it. There was my husband standing looking at me and his sleeping body and there was I thinking that his spirit had left his body. Later I was to learn that this was indeed a case of my husband being away in his astral body while his physical slept next to me."

I have selected a few interesting examples from the many letters which I have received about this inner personality, and its ability to move out of physical focus, as it were, and yet be connected with the physical body by a mysterious hierarchy of energy systems.

In the account of two personal experiences which I am about to narrate it will be seen that the two mediumistic individuals claimed to have had vivid memories of being out of their bodies after falling asleep.

While living in Cape Town I was asked by a colleague to see a female alcoholic who was an artist. She modelled some excellent heads of ancient Bushmen and several specimens of native tribes. Her work was most impressive as to detailed production of the features characterising and individualising the personality. At the time of my visit she had just recovered from fourteen days of almost alcoholic stuper but was presentable, rational and dignified in speech and bearing.

Towards the end of the consultation I noticed a planchette on top of the wardrobe. I asked her about her experiences with the planchette, and she told me how at times when in need of inspiration she would put her hand on the planchette and receive what she thought was automatic writing. On occasions this would be a description of some head, characterised by the expression of some particular emotion or trait of personality in the facial expression, such as slyness, cunning, wickedness or naive innocence. With this would come a mental picture which she would then model.

What interested me especially in this account of her experiences was her story that she had often come to herself in a state which was not a dream, but a vital logical objective experience of visiting some queer or outstanding character often in the far-away Kalahari desert land, where the Bushmen roamed in their tribal traditional way.

She was sure that her spirit left her body and roamed to gain impressions and mental material for her livelihood. I discovered that her bouts of drinking were precipitated by an inborn recurrent depression. I was about to leave her rather lonely little cottage, where she lived with an old coloured servant when an impulse seized me and made me ask her to put her fingers on the planchette with mine. Within moments of our fingers lightly touching the planchette it started rushing wildly all over the large sheet of drawing paper.

I felt that she might be pushing it as I certainly was completely passive. Somewhat annoyed and visibly offended she denied that she exercised any pressure in any direction. The planchette however continued whirling round and round as if caught up in some maelstrom. She said that it was gathering power. Then the circular movements became slower and slower and suddenly it began to write. I could not see what it was writing and she was looking at the ceiling and not at the planchette.

Abruptly it stopped, as if with a movement of triumph. We looked at the writing. There it was distinct, bold and clear in Afrikaans : "Moenie bang wees vir die dood nie." (Don't be afraid of death) and then the signature with each letter distinctly and neatly formed—"Piet de Villiers Moll." I was to say the least dumbfounded for a moment.

Dr. Piet de Villiers Moll was a well-known Cape Town orthopaedic surgeon who was killed on safari a few days before my meeting with this lady. He was a friend of mine and the night before he left on a big-game hunt somewhere in Central Africa we were together at a social function, where incidentally he and I discussed parapsychological phenomena. He admitted unfamiliarity with the subject and also a resistance of mind to accept the reality of parapsychology.

I immediately questioned her about the late Dr. Moll, but she disclaimed all knowledge of him, and what was more she had not heard of his death, as she had no radio and had not seen a newspaper for the previous few days since she was at that time in an alcoholic stuperous sleep. I did not mention this experience to any member of the late Dr. Moll's family but retained this impressive and unique memory. The significance of the sentence typified the way he would have expressed himself once he discovered that he was not dead. He was a concise dynamic and extremely witty personality, as dexterous with his tongue as with his healing hands.

During the few years that followed I often thought of Pietie Moll as he was known to his friends and colleagues, and I was one of the prime movers in establishing a fund for orthopaedic work in his name. Then came 1936 and I was in Queenstown. There I met a colleague, the late Dr. Winter who had a deep interest in psychic research. I told him about Moll and the planchette.

Then one day I was called to see a white female patient in her twenties. She had an abscess in her groin and I arranged for the surgeon to open it, while I would give her a whiff of ether. While preparing her for this minor operation she asked me to put her to sleep without the anaesthetic. She responded quickly and was a good hypnotic subject. Thereafter I saw her several times and learned that she had recovered from a severe depressive condition. She was completely rational and intelligent.

She told me about a peculiar dream in which she knew that her body was sleeping in the bed, while she was talking to a soldier who was killed in World War 1. He came from her home-town and knew her as a little girl. He always made a fuss of her and brought her sweets. The first time she met him in her dreams he appeared in uniform and his head was bandaged, while his uniform was bespattered with mud. Thereafter he changed, and would meet her in a dreamworld place with gardens, playing fountains and beautiful flowers. His body was clothed but in a soft white material. She somehow only remembered his face. The impression however was quite distinct that she was travelling in a form which was not her body' because it was light and airy. He told her that he had been killed in Flanders, and that he did not know that he was dead at first until he thought it strange that he could walk through barbed wire. The world which he took her to in through her sleep was his home.

He said that the two of them belonged to the same spiritual family, and that he was her guardian. I instructed her to observe all that she could during her sleep travels, and to ask him to tell her what the world was like where he was living. I discussed this with Dr. Winter and invited him to join me in investigating this girl's mind, because it was just possible that she was making up these stories to maintain our interest and to be of some importance.

To our surprise she related a dream in which her guide took her to see a place very much like the earth, except that the colours were more vivid. The flowers seemed to make their colours if one looked at them and desired them to be beautiful. She saw towns and villages but the other people appeared to be working with their imaginations. Her friend told her that if I put her to sleep he would bring someone who wanted to demonstrate something.

Dr. Winter and I decided to try this experiment. We took her to my study where we would be undisturbed. She was made to lie down on a couch and we took her heart rate and blood pressure. Her heart was beating round about 90 to 84 beats per minute and her blood pressure was 136/80. We chatted for a while and then I induced a deep hypnotic trance.

I told her that since someone unknown to us wanted to use her mind, she would repress all thoughts from her consciousness which were not in keeping with our purpose. Her mind would become refined and extremely sensitive to thoughts coming from beyond this world, in fact from those known as the dead. She would be able to talk and act out any impression which she received. In the meantime she would await in serene calmness what was to come.

I would like to digress here to mention a skill in whistling which the late Dr. Moll often displayed at dances. He was able to whistle out of the corner of his mouth with hardly any distortion of the normal appearance of his mouth. This peculiar ability combined with his charming and entertaining personality was often most amusing to his dancing partner when his facial expression remained mask-like.

Now to return to our experiment. The subject went into a deep hypnotic sleep, and for a while all was quiet. The cuff of the sphygmamonometer was retained on her arm, as we wanted to study the pulse rate and blood pressure should any phenomenon occur. The moments passed. Her respiration became slow. Her body started to twist and turn while her head remained in one place as if held there, and the body only moved in attempts which appeared as if it wanted to loosen the neck or pull it away. At this stage and in spite of the movement the pulse rate dropped from 90 to 56 beats per minute. The movement of the arm with the cuff made it impossible to obtain the blood pressure reading.

As this strange twisting and turning of the body from the shoulders downwards continued, we noticed that her face became congested. It had a decided bluish tint. My colleague became concerned and feared that she was going to have a convulsion. He thought that we should terminate the trance. I was adamant however that even if she had a convulsion it would not be fatal. There followed a few more spasmodic movements and then she was quiet and relaxed. Blood pressure 100/80, pulse rate 40. Respiration slow.

As we sat looking at her the bluish tint was replaced by a paleness, and for a moment I shared my colleague's anxiety. Then she smiled, and there before our eyes she whistled out of the corner of her mouth. A sharp clear whistling sound and Dr. Winter looked at me in utter amazement. His gentle clear big eyes spoke volumes, for I had told him about this peculiar skill of Dr. Moll. To others this would appear no more than a mere description of a mannerism of a friend, but to me at that moment it was the recognition of personality, and the realization of an astonishing reality; the same feeling as when my wife's mother announced her departure from this world and kept her promise.

The young lady had an extremely poor Afrikaans vocabulary, and her pronunciation was equally bad. In fact she did not know sufficient Afrikaans to conduct a simple conversation. After she had whistled and smiled she spoke in clear, well pronounced Afrikaans : 'Hello, ek het vir julle 'n demonstrasie gelewer van my ontrekking uit u wêreld. Jy sal my eerste kommunikasie deur middel van die planchette onthou. Dit was al wat ek op daardie oomblik kon doen om bewys te lewer van my ontwakking. Nou het ek die geleentheid geneem om my vertrek deur die dood te herlewe, die ontbinding van my gees. Laat haar slaap en vanself wakker word want sy was dieper as die gewone hipnotiese trans. Mit segen aufwedersehn."

The English version of the communication is as follows : "Hello I have just given you a demonstration of my withdrawal from your world. You will remember my first communication by means of the planchette. It was all I could manage at that time to give proof of my awakening over here. Now I have taken the opportunity to relive the process of my death. The release of my spiritual self. Let her sleep and wake up by herself because she was deeper than the usual hypnotic trance. With blessings—till we meet again."

Did this young lady who was undoubtedly mediumistic read my thoughts in the same manner that Solomon Daba did at his seance dance? I can only say that I did not expect Dr. Moll to communicate. Her behaviour and the extreme slowing of the pulse rate and respiration indicated that her organism was being used to give a reproduction of the event of his death. I learned later that his neck had been pinned between the door and the body of the truck, which overturned while he was swerving in the attempt to avoid a native child who ran across the road.

I do not know the post mortem findings, but if his neck had been pinned by the door of the truck and he had lived for a while then the twisting and turning of the body were movements which he could have made before he lost consciousness. But above all do I consider and so did Dr. Winter that the whistle out of the corner of her mouth was the most genuine evidence of his personality, much more so than the subject's speech in Afrikaans. I tried on several occasions even under hypnosis to make the young lady reproduce that whistle and she was quite incapable of doing so.

There was another aspect of that hypnotic trance conversation, namely his last words in German. This young lady knew no German whereas Dr. Moll was a graduate of a German University and spoke the language fluently. The year before this experiment I had returned from a short visit to German psychiatric institutions and having a limited German vocabulary made use of the opportunity to speak German to my friend Dr. Winter, especially in front of hospital patients when we did not want to be understood. It could thus be that we provided certain telepathic conditions, but the meaningfulness of the words "mit segen aufwedersehn" came to me a few years later when I learned of the sudden death of my friend Dr. Winter.

The hypnotic trance experiment was really done with the object of ascertaining the nature of her dream travels. We were interested in the astral personality, because we felt that it held the key to the secret relations between mind and matter, and especially of the faculties such as clairvoyance, telepathy and precognition.

We thought that the one who wanted to communicate, as she had been informed by her soldier guardian friend, would give us information of the astral plane, and explain whether her dream pictures were actual astral scenes or mere products of her imagination and perhaps demonstrate ectoplasm. Instead of finding an answer to these questioning thoughts Dr. Pietie Moll came, and by means of Afrikaans and German produced evidence which candidly was beyond the mental ability of the subject at that time. But apart from all this impressive evidence was the individual characteristic and skill, the capability to whistle out of the corner of his mouth. Many people might be able to perform a similar feat, but Dr. Pietie Moll knew how much his whistling always amused and intrigued me.

We made several attempts by means of the hypnotic trance to provide opportunities for Moll to communicate again, but no mind claiming to be his ever made contact with us again. Instead we obtained some interesting descriptions of life on the astral from the soldier friend of her dream world.

CHAPTER X

THE SIGNIFICANCE OF PSYCHIC PHENOMENA

The experiences of people who have found themselves outside their physical bodies have left us with a premise for deep thinking. They have for instance solved the problem of the relation between body and mind in so far that their experience has shown that mind in reality belongs not to body as we know it but to this inner or astral personality with its thoughts, memories and emotions.

Apparently then the non recognition of this astral personality has left the philosophers groping around in sterile ideas, when we compare their conclusions with the living experiences of men and women. Bertrand Russel in "What I believe" states : "What we call our thoughts seem to depend upon the organization of tracks in the brain in the same way in which journeys depend on railways. The energy used in thinking seems to have a chemical origin," and "We also cannot suppose that an individual's thinking survives bodily death, since that destroys the organization of the brain and dissipates the energy which uses the brain tracks."

Here then we have the conclusions of one of the world's great philosophers. But when we place this type of reasoning alongside of the evidence which I have collected we are impressed by the limitation of vision and consciousness which the leading and most brilliant intellects of our day display when dealing with matters of a metaphysical nature. We observe that thought is considered as energy having a chemical origin. This concession should rightly equally include the recognition that energy is not only indestructible, but that it also possesses the property of transformation.

More interesting still is the accepted fact that there is no fundamental difference between energy and matter. They are indeed the same according to modern physics. One could add that when it is in the form of matter, energy is locked up. Now the human organism including its brain and thought tracks is finally nothing else, but a form of organized energy. One can best understand this organization as a spectrum of life with different wavebands and frequency rates of energy vibration.

Man's evolution of consciousness could therefore be his sole aim and purpose and this evolution could consist of a process of transformation or shedding of forms of energy, and there is no reason why the progress of his Ego or Self from one plane of existence to another should not according to the spectrum of life on a particular plane be clothed in an organization of energy which we could call a body or a vehicle of expression.

We know that energy continues to exist according to the law of conservation of energy. Therefore if this law and its operation make man a form of organized energy on earth, why should it not do the same with energy at a higher frequency rate of the spectrum of life for instance as it apparently does on the astral plane. It is indeed illogical to accept these facts about energy, as well as the fact that man is organized energy, and then deny that this truth and fundamental principle should not apply to an astral being. When our thoughts follow this line of reason and logic then we should have little theoretical difficulty in accepting the reality of the astral personality.

We can of course conclude that our modern philosophers have not devoted their unprejudiced intellects to this vast field of parapsychology, including decades of the findings of psychic research. They have based their thoughts on the discoveries of science, but science will be the first to acknowledge that it has abstracted what concerned and served its purpose, and the object it had in view, and that its scientific concepts were designed for certain purposes and interests. The conclusion which this fact forces on our minds is that science deals not with the whole of reality, but only with a partial aspect of reality. In its present stage of evolution it is wearing blinkers. But men of science will not assert, I am sure, that what science has ignored in life is less real and less important than what it has accepted, pursued, discovered and applied.

Once intellectual and scientific men agree with the evidence that man possesses an inner component of a more refined substance known as his astral personality, which the process of death completely liberates from the physical body, and which after this separation continues to retain mental faculties and a consciousness, then really it should not be impossible to associate and attribute psychic functions such as clairvoyance, telepathy, precognition and psychokinesis to this inner energy organization of man known as the astral.

Physical man reveals a fundamental law of his nature, and that is his hierarchy of structure and function. By means of correspondence we can perceive and understand the same hierarchical law of life rising from a brain consciousness to an astral, and then to a pure psychical degree, as steps of the abstract hierarchical law of consciousness.

Even then in the unseen world of man there is a correspondence in this hierarchical character of his life. This conception should serve as a valid guide to our thought especially where it is difficult to form a picture of these abstract regions of life. It is hence of profound interest to observe and accept as factual that the study of physical man reveals clear evidence of a system of hierarchy not only of his brain cell arrangement and function, but of his instincts and drives. It has besides its physical reality its mental correspondence. Now, when we turn to the supernormal evidence of psychic phenomena supporting survival after death, we are enabled to understand this hierarchical law as a system underlying man's spiritual evolution and the development of higher degrees of consciousness.

The evidence for the existence of ectoplasm for instance is indisputable. This energy system comes into being and becomes solid and then vanishes like the electron. This fact shows higher forms of energy beyond the gross physical appearance of man. So here as a matter of physical demonstration we have an ectoplasmic energy system which undergoes transformation before our eyes from the objective into the abstract. Evidence of this nature taken in conjunction with the hierarchical law of life helps us to understand how life produces beings of an inner energy organization as astral, psychical or spiritual beings according to our nomenclature.

Astral projection establishes the fact that the physical personality has an inner or non physical complementary personality. The latter is composed of the psychological and emotional equipment which we develop in response to the stimulations of this physical world. The astral personality is hence a preservation or a survival of these characteristics of the person. It is an inner organization of the being with a finer energy substance.

But we must not conclude that because the energy organization of the astral body is of a higher order in the hierarchy of life than the physical, that anyone who enters the astral automatically attains a higher sense of ethics, aesthetics and spiritual knowledge. A person living in the flesh can have a consciousness of much higher development in its comprehension of psychic reality, than a discarnate being existing on the astral plane. This difference is the result of the capacity for development of the consciousness of man, and depends perhaps mostly on the luminescence of the psyche which in the final analysis can be no other than the individuality of the personality.

Consciousness is defined in psychological terms as "a character belonging to certain processes or events in the living organism, which must be regarded as unique, and therefore indefinable in terms of anything else, but which can perhaps best be described as a view of these processes or events from the inside. The individual is as it were inside what is happening." The significance of the above definition is the emphasis on within, the inside, the inner view and the position of being inside what is happening, and above all our utter inability to define it in terms of anything else comprised within our highest knowledge of today. It has no counterpart in our physical domain.

The world of medicine is associated with a system of organs or a hierarchy of the central nervous system. In this system consciousness is said to be integrated at various nerve cell levels, and is said to be dependent on reverberating circuits of energy flowing between the grey matter of the brain and the grey matter of the midbrain as well as the brain stem and the spinal cord.

Consciousness is therefore considered to be associated with the activity of the cells of the grey matter covering the brain, and this activity is again dependent on the sensory impulses coming into the brain from our sight, touch, smell, hearing and taste as well as temperatures and so on, including impulses of nerve currents from our inner bodily organs.

But this does not complete the picture, because science has discovered that sensory nerve currents reaching the grey matter or cortex cannot by themselves maintain consciousness, but that there is an upflow or radiation of nervous energy from the midbrain which activates the cells of the grey matter, and furthermore that consciousness cannot be present in the brain if this mysterious radiation of life energy from the hypothalamus is not operating. It establishes a central dominance, which actually controls the amount of stimulation which comes from the senses and their nerves. This therefore forms a regulating system, and is a dynamic consciousness, a reality force which is expressed by life.

As it flows into many channels to millions of little batteries known as nerve cells it causes them to be in a state of vigilance, which is triggered into content such as images, as these sense impressions arrive from the outside in the brain. In other words one can compare this upflow or radiation of energy forming consciousness, as the current coming from the main to the radio, and the impulses from the sense organs can be compared with the broadcast. There can be no content, no voice or music, no reception in fact unless the current from the main operates the radio.

This little peep into the energy systems employed by brain consciousness, or better still the sensory intellectual consciousness of man, shows us that psychic life is not a flicker of consciousness travelling over the brain, or a by-product of brain cell activity. It has at the back of it a purpose, and this purposefulness cannot be dissociated from intelligence. The latter therefore must be a component of all living substance however rudimentary or minute its flicker of consciousness. Hence consciousness should be understood in no other light than as an expression of life, by means of which we view our world of experience from within, while we are sustained by a current from the cosmic main and power-station of life.

Man is composed of billions of cells, each one has been called an amazing little chemical factory, and yet a living entity, and hence it too must possess a modicum of consciousness and instinctive intelligence. Each little cell is no more than a mass of jelly surrounded by a membrane with a nucleus inside and near its centre. The moment the nucleus is removed the cell dies. Inside the cell are minute particles of living matter called proteins and in the whole of the cell granules can be seen streaming hither and thither, floating in currents of life. Some times they push through the membrane and protrude the cell's substance like the ectoplasmic protrusions from a trance medium.

I have often wondered whether these mysterious properties of the cell are not the energy substance of ectoplasm? The cells are of many different species and although their membranes limit them these do not prevent contact with their fellows. They breathe and take in nourishment and discharge waste material. There are other cells always on the prowl throughout one's body, and the moment a cell is sick or dying or enfeebled by age these prowling cells attack it and destroy it by eating or engulfing the dead cell as their nourishment.

Each cell behaves as though it has a purpose or a desire to fulfill its task. It is difficult therefore to deny it a little bit of intelligence and consciousness. From a newspaper I recently learned of Dr. Eccles an English scientist who advanced a theory on memory. Dr. Eccles believes that nervous stimuli supplied to the brain by the sense organs circle continuously in "neuronal oscillating circuits" and are available as memory as long as the circuits remain active. Now this is precisely what the electronic brain does : it stores information in an oscillating circuit.

Then Professor Glees also did work on this theory of Dr. Eccles and he said :

"Any experience causes a flow of electrons to the nerve cells, as part of nervous stimulation. This alters the chemical equilibrium inside the cell. The information proteins are continuously synthesized anew to replace those decomposed in the process of ordinary protein metabolism. In these curious archives everything is continuously copied afresh, which is not a very economical method but the safest one in view of the short-lived protein material."

The protein of the cell on this theory carries the impression or image brought by the senses while the circuits of electronic currents flow from the hypothalamus of the brain. The protein like the electron disappears and is replaced by a new one. This recording hence takes place in hidden activities of brain cells, and since memories and intelligence operate in the astral it can be assumed that the ectoplasmic energy of the cell receives it from the protein circuit and transmits it to the astral, and so the astral consciousness develops its store of earthly memories, ideas and interests.

Now memory is a psychic retentivity, a psychic quality of existence, and cannot come into being without consciousness. Hence the little cell as an individual shares in this energy radiation which forms the self-awareness of man, with its qualities of appreciating, perceiving and remembering. Man's intellect however is for the practical purpose of living and concerns the brain, but what is registered in the brain by the flash of a highly charged protein is simultaneously recorded in the astral substance of the brain.

Behind all this and viewing these recorded happenings and events is the Self. We know it exists but we do not know what it is, and astonishing as it may seem, it is impossible for one to know the true self by means of thought, because thoughts are after all only emanations or radiations of the self. One is therefore because of this hierarchy of consciousness in all its different degrees really prevented from knowing the self as a whole. The thoughts are only relevant to the vehicle of energy, which the physical or the astral self employs to express itself.

The main power of the self is its consciousness, which in physical man plays upon the brain cells like a spray of water from the fountain of life in the hypothalamus of the brain. This consciousness gives the self the view from within, and this feeling of awareness requires the existence of other things, besides the self, as viewer of life's panorama, without the existence of other objects and beings it will have no identity or self consciousness, and yet all our ghost and spirit stories reveal self consciousness. Hence they move in worlds of other beings as well as themselves.

The self is hence identical with consciousness and thought is its relation to its surroundings or plane of existence whether physical or astral. One can picture consciousness to have levels like the floors of a huge skyscraper. The Ego reaches a floor, and has a medium of expression by means of the nature of the substance of that floor, and it looks out of a window and sees a view and then its relative consciousness forms thoughts of that view.

The sensory intellect belongs to the lowest storeys of the self-building. The Self or Ego behaves like an elevator which stops at different floors for the evolution of consciousness. It experiences knowledge at each level, because to be conscious is to know.

Cognition is hence a means whereby the Self at different stages individualizes itself.

The Self and its consciousness evolves after death by a constant process of learning and adaptation, because we have seen these fundamental principles operating on the astral. The consciousness can be earthbound by its former wishes and desires and so the Self will not progress merely because it has undergone the change of death. It requires the development of other qualities of mind as well.

The astral can only promote a higher consciousness if the individual has the capacity to envisage an abstract existence, and has at some time or other within his secret thoughts experienced the emotional moments of wonder at the vast unknown ahead. Consciousness does not seem to be in a hurry for it grows and expands by laws of understanding while it is nourished by the desire to know and the power to feel a sympathy for life.

There is no need to attempt to jump the gap of the ultimate reality. Our experience in psychic phenomena has shown that a substantial existence lies in close proximity to this life, in the nature of the astral plane. It is much wiser for us to study this abstract reality and obtain as much knowledge as possible about it while we are in this life. We can study this next phase with precision once the right mediums are available, for ectoplasm and materializations may in this era bring the immediate next phase nearer for our comprehension of some of the impulses which we feel.

Indeed the logic of the astral is our next reality. The other storeys of the building of individual life are too high and perhaps too far among the spiritual clouds for most people. Our consciousness should first be prepared by systematized thought to move from confused thought and feeling to higher goals. He whose mind is prepared to progress from the astral can never be anchored to earth by a limitation of consciousness.

The unique function of our sensory intellectual consciousness has been shown to be only one form of psychic awareness on the lowest rungs of the hierarchy of man's invisible organizations of energy. Apart from this man has been able to produce evidence of a peculiar degree of consciousness known as mystic experience. It can be expected that scientific psychology will discount any experience known as mystic, for the simple reason that these states of awareness are dissociated from the logic presented to the brain by the sensory intellectual consciousness of our daily lives.

These mystic states are too abstract for scientific psychology, besides they seem to consist of feeling rather than perception. Nevertheless scientific psychology cannot ignore the evidence in favour of psi phenomena especially the researches of Dr. J. B. Rhine and his co-workers at Duke's University. These researches bear ample evidence that since these psychic faculties do not require sense organs, they imply the existence of a form of consciousness which operates without the assistance of time or space.

This transcendental form of consciousness however although rare cannot be dismissed, because since we have such mental functions as clairvoyance, telepathy and precognition all showing clear purposive directions of thought, we find it reasonable to view such manifestations as revelations of higher attainments of the Ego.

In these states people have felt a oneness of the hidden energies which the sensory intellectual degree of consciousness is unable to grasp. The mystic experience seems to view objects and differentiated entities as forms of energy and not material things. Actually the mystic consciousness seems to tell us the same story as physics namely that mass and energy are the same thing only the mystic experience reveals the energy as the most dominant impression.

This mystic impression in the mind is one of wholeness, sublimity, beauty and giveness. The feelings take the place of the senses, and constitute the very essence of existence, and so can hardly ever be described in words. It reveals the inner life of certain degrees of the cosmos. These emotional moments are flashes of feeling illuminating the unpenetrated future of life, revealing a unity which is wonderfully vast, and all-embracing, while at the same moment exalted in glory and grandeur.

This mystic experience cannot be described otherwise than as being the acme of self consciousness. We see evidence of this self consciousness in astral projection, when the self in astral form can stand outside his physical body, and be conscious that it is his body, and yet travel away by means of wish, will and desire ignoring brick walls and doors for he does not need their resistance to his passage to convince himself of his identity and existence. He has found his reality in the consciousness of his astral self.

Perhaps those who have had these transcendental mystic experiences have reached the depths of cosmic existence which revealed in a glimpse the higher hierarchical levels of the soul's vision of its world. It seems as though the emotional quality of wonder which blossomed in our early childhood years finds its ultimate goal in a mystic experience. Should one analyse this sense of wonder one will find that it is always tinged with some feeling of veneration.

Wonder appears to be necessary somehow to prepare man's

mind for the eternal truth and seems to constitute the germinal steps towards mystic feelings. A mystic experience cannot be attained by thinking or reasoning—it is something which comes upon one. Indeed it is consciousness without thinking of any known thing. It simply supersedes one's rational consciousness. It hovers far above and so obliterates for the moment sensations, images, emotions and ideas of action. This is where all words fail.

Those who have had these experiences have left us the impression that they had seen separate and distinct entities, but were at the same time tremendously and overwhelmingly conscious of a basic unity underlying their existence as being mere constituents of an unfathomable whole, whose energy organization is their final unity. This has remained the lasting and most exalted realization and feeling of a mystic experience.

One night while attending a patient during a confinement on a lonely farm, and while waiting for the slow progress of the woman in labour, the farmer and I talked of many things as we drank coffee into the small hours of the morning. It was then that he told me of a strange experience which came upon him one day high up in the mountains.

The phenomena of nature, the flowers in the spring, the things which grew and the cascading little waterfalls as well as the lazy drifting clouds always inspired him in a mysterious manner to think poetically. Sometimes he would write his poems down but always the melody of words and their hidden meanings would fade once he laboured intellectually at clothing his feelings with words.

On this particular afternoon he sat on one of the highest peaks having just come from his sheep station beyond the mountain range. He looked down over the valley and the vineyards below, while up there he sat in absolute silence, under a sky that was almost thick with its blueness and again he felt an urge to express his appreciation of the reverence of that moment. There was something within him that wanted to come out, indeed a strange desire to reach out into space and feel it and interpret it as a poetical reality.

Then while immersed in this emotion of reverence, he looked at a piece of quartz which he held in his hand, and as he looked at it and its glistening gold-like speckles, suddenly an intense illumination engulfed him. He saw millions of little stars with rainbow rings streaming from them in place of the piece of quartz, and he felt his consciousness enter into every particle belonging to an infinite whole, while his being was buoyant with intense delight for he knew at that moment that he had looked into God. And then in a flash it was gone, but the memory remained as a relic of his celestial soul.

After this supernormal experience, this peep into eternity as it were, he was naturally puzzled and his first concern was whether there was some abnormality in the function of his brain. He remembered a servant he once had who had fits and who saw visions and became exalted before an attack. He being an intelligent rational being became genuinely anxious that all the beatitude might perhaps have been the result of an abnormal delusional brain condition.

Anyway this happened five years before he communicated his extraordinary experience to me and he has never had a recurrence or anything in the nature of a disturbance of consciousness since that day. In the absence of any irrational episode in his life and any history suggestive of epilepsy I came to the conclusion that his was a true mystic state of consciousness.

Experiences of this nature are unusual if not quite foreign to our mundane existence, nevertheless it would be quite unwise to push them aside as nonsense, and to deny them the significance of a deeper insight, especially when no psychiatrical abnormality can be discovered in behaviour and history. On the other hand should we take them seriously we are driven to admit the occasional emergence and swamping of consciousness by the hidden faculties of the psyche.

The mystic experience although so profoundly abstract and different from our sensory intellectual consciousness, is not so unique and so impossible to understand once we look around for other non-sensory forms of knowledge. Most of us who work at intellectual tasks must admit that at some time or other we have received impressions or ideas which did not come from the outside world via our senses. This process of what I shall call intellectual intuition, is a definite cognitive faculty of the human mind. And yet it is a manner of comprehension, or almost revelation of knowledge which somehow provides a complete answer to one's mental struggles or enquiries.

I have always called this intellectual intuition "influx" for it seems to come as a supercharge of mind which sorts out all one's misunderstandings in an effortless manner only after you have laboured at some obtruse idea, and in that moment one appreciates the problem directly, there is no devious pathway, and the truth is immediately grasped, because all the parts have taken up their harmonious relations and their correct positions to present the idea of the whole to one's consciousness.

These moments in which man is taken out of his depths by means of mind, and the world of ideas, clearly show that they are glimpses of other regions to which thought could have access. For most of us all experience comes via the sensory intellectual consciousness. But this plane of consciousness is unobtrusively invaded by the provisions of the intellectual intuitive consciousness, and the latter is treated without its warranted significance as a "hunch" and taken for granted without any inquiry as to its source, motive and purpose.

But when we view this picture we perceive the correspondence of the law of hierarchy and the next stage of understanding gives us the astral consciousness which seems to separate itself from the sensory intellectual awareness of man and portrays such faculties as clairvoyance, telepathy and precognition. These psychic powers probably produced the intellectual intuition or hunch, but did so as a presentation of ideas as part of a completed whole, and not as supernormal forms of perception. If then we follow this conception of the hierarchy we ultimately come to the rarest of all namely the mystic experience or awareness of the soul's Ego.

Approaching man's mind from this aspect brings us to the realization that the psyche of man is an archive within whose recesses are hidden powerful means of comprehension not only of our physical world, but understanding of more and more abstract planes of life in the path of destiny. Perhaps these inner visions come to the surface of consciousness because of the secret powers of temperament, interest and the ability to feel and think in terms of the abstract.

Perhaps we are so preoccupied with our sense impressions, that we are from moment to moment unaware of the meaningfulness which these higher extrasensory and even mystic seepages from the soul of man give to his sensory world of ideas and actions. Perhaps we are not even aware of the gaps and disconnections in our thoughts and sense impressions which are continually being filled in and connected as trains of thought by higher and higher means of inflow or influx.

There is a responsiveness in us, indeed a hidden and endless ability to resonate with situations and stimulations. We see this when music, beauty and aesthetic influences call forth feelings from other strata of the Ego where it expresses its particular world of ideas and meanings, and each serves as a stage on the way to the ultimate truth which at times is felt as a mystic experience of total intunement with cosmic reality.

This unique function of consciousness defined as a view from within is nevertheless the life power of the Ego or Self. The sensory intellectual consciousness seems to consist of a field of force or aura, and into this aura new ideas are born every moment, while others enter from other persons. But we should not leave out of consideration the dynamic radiations of life in terms of endocrine glands and body biochemistry forming the temperamental qualities of personality.

All these energy systems bring about electromagnetic charges in the aura of man and are known as the powers of instincts, wishes and beliefs, not excluding fanatical, overdetermined and obsessive ideas. How many of these are inherited is difficult to say. Could man inherit a race memory for instance? Anyway this aura of man must be a battleground for many conflicting drives and motivations. Hence it is man's task to gain an insight into his sensory intellectual life, while still on earth, otherwise he will have to await the results of the laws of monotony or exhaustion of repetition of the same thought and action on the astral plane before a new adjustment is possible to a higher degree of consciousness.

Having examined some of these strange phenomena of man's psychic life, and the mysterious powers of his nonsensory experience including the various and different manifestations of levels of consciousness, one stands before the question : How did life originate on this planet? And how did these complex and wonderful organizations of energy systems come about to produce the dynamic personality of man?

Julian Huxley in his book *Evolution in Action* in dealing with this question of the origin of life, states : "To start with life is not a thing, a separate entity. It is a word used to describe the properties and activities of living substance, as observed in animals and plants, and their basic distinguishing property is their capacity for self-production. It in turn appears to be linked with complex chemical molecules in which nucleic acid is combined with a protein."

One observes that this erudite and brilliant intellect has been confined to one perspective in his view of life. He goes on : "There are only three possible alternatives as regards the origin of living substance on earth. Either it is supernormally created : or it was brought to the earth from some other place in the universe in the interior of a meteorite : or it was produced naturally out of less complicated substances."

He dismissed the first suggestion of creation as divine interference, and considers it illogical and unnecessary. He points out that living substance consists of the same matter as lifeless substance : it transacts its operations according to the same general rules. "There is no trace of any special vital force which can be detected or measured. Both the inorganic and the organic world are built of the same matter and work by means of the same energy."

He comes to the conclusion that living substance evolved out of the non living. He considers this the only hypothesis consistent with scientific continuity. He also considers that because spontaneous generation does not occur now is no evidence that it did not occur at some earlier stage of the development of this planet: "When conditions in the cosmic test tube were extremely different." He considers that life started from the property possessed by carbon of linking its atoms. He continues :"It must be confessed however that the actual process is still conjectural; all we know is that living substance must have developed soon after the first rocks of the geological strata were laid down, and that this was somewhere about two thousand million years ago."

We observe that the scientific theory as propounded by Julian Huxley implies that life came forth out of inorganic matter. He does not seem to realize that this idea is more miraculous than the metaphorical language Genesis conveys of the origin of life. He admits however that this scientific theory of the beginning of life is conjectural—that means that it is a judgment formed from incomplete evidence. In other words it is a convenient surmise or guess because of ignorance.

Spontaneous generation meant originally that life came from some putrifying matter. Huxley has substituted for this the miracle of the carbon atom producing a gene as the first form of life here. Lord Kelvin thought that life germs reached us from some other planet. We observe however that no higher psychic values or non physical states of life are conceived of in these scientific definitions of origins. Candidly Huxley's idea is more a blind faith and not anything based on scientific fact to assume that life started from inorganic matter and that life is therefore a product of matter.

Hence when we study the theories of the origin of life on this planet and we bear in mind the supernormal evidence of psychic research, as well as the experiences of people which I have recorded, then we must realize that the scientific theory is hardly capable of dealing with life as through the supernormal, we have come to know it. Indeed there is no scientific theory worthy of one's intellectual respect. And not only does this apply to the origin of life, but it equally applies to the origin of the personality of Homo Sapiens.

One comes to the question that because of these totally inadequate and conjectural theories of origin whether it is wise for us to accept these theories as an act of faith, especially the one of man's evolution from a carbon atom and eventually from a primitive organism in the slime of a cooling earth?

Scientific men point with confidence to their findings of geological records, but these have been interpreted in accordance with the general theory propounded by Darwin. Indeed the picture of the fossils were clothed and formed by means of artistic creative imagination to conform to a so-called continuous chain from primate to man as thought out by Darwin. One is entitled to ask : is this really how it all happened or are the deductions merely fulfilling the requirements of a theory?

So on the theory of geological deposits Homo Sapiens is a latecomer to this world having been preceded by his ape-like ancestors. All this fits well into the Darwinian concept, but what has always been of interest to me was that Wallace the co-inventor with Darwin of the theory of natural selection had thoughts about the incompatibility of this theory with the idea that man has an inner consciousness and soul. Wallace however squared his conscience by thinking that mind and soul were specially created for man.

It does appear as if the men of science are at times unaware of the miraculous claims, which seem to rival even those of the old testament. Wallace felt the need to accept this inner psychic life of man, because if there had been a gradual progression from ape-like ancestor to modern man then such an historical process must raise the question as to when during this process this creature acquired a human psyche or soul, capable of sensory intellectual consciousness, intellectual intuition, psi faculties, and finally the capacity for a mystic experience?

The geological deposits do not adequately reveal to us a correspondence of external expression of such a psychic evolution in the behaviour and conscious values of this missing link creature. Hence we are entitled to conclude with all respect for those who have laboured in the interest of science that even the smooth flow of the Darwinian theory has in actual fact not bridged the gulf between man and his nearest ape-like forerunners.

Also there is the conception that our evolution from primates is a faith based on the idea that fossil men showed different degrees of intelligence. But even this theory of progressive evolution of intelligence remains steeped in suppositions and surmises. One does not deny that humble forms of life have rudimentary intelligence and consciousness however rigid and instinctively confined to certain activities, but the observed facts do not support a continuous process of growth and expansion of intelligence as a dynamic force through a range of creatures from a carbon atom to spiritual man.

If the emergence of a consciousness and self-realization as found in man came along a long line of descent from perhaps a carbon atom and then a speck of jelly in primordial slimy water, one would expect to find the steps of the species through which it came not in fossil correspondences, but also in the products of thought.

Because of the all-convincing purposefulness of life as we know it, one finds it difficult to accept the scientific idea of the origin of life as an emergence by sheer chance out of inorganic matter. By conjectures, models and surmises and creative purposeful imagination science has utilised fossil remains and made Darwin's theory an objective museum fact, and so gave reality values to the sensory intellectual conclusions of mind as the last word on the origin of man.

But if the true reality of man is non-physical, and if the physical body is merely the primary and most external vehicle for the evolution of his consciousness, then the theory of evolution does not meet the case. Because the moment the mind of the intelligent and literate man chooses an approach to life, which grants reality values to inner degrees of personality, known by such names as ethereal-self, astral-self, psyche or soul, then the conflict on this plane between the accepted theory of evolution and the inner man, becomes one which intelligence of the highest order must face. It becomes a challenge of man's need for knowledge.

I recently came across a book "Man, God and Magic" by Ivar Lissner. He states after careful examination of the evidence and quoting the views of leading thinkers "that we know of no instance where one form has gradually changed into another," and "the famous Dresden naturalist and theologian Arthur Neuberg has pointed out that a dog's embryo cell can never produce anything but a dog, but children at school are still being taught that long ago man was an amoeba, then a fish, then a reptile and so on."

He quotes O. Speelbeck : "We do not know how man came into being," and "Man is a unique and extraordinary phenomenon; in Overhage's words "an event far transcending all organic evolutions." He goes on : "There are certain facts which cast doubt on the whole theory of man's upward development and evolution by stages from Anthropoid via the Neanderthalian to the Sapiens type. We owe our knowledge of these facts to American, British, French and German scholars, men like Leaky, Connolly, Oakley, Howell, Montagu, Remane and Overhage."

The evidence collected by Ivar Lissner produces proof that Homo Sapiens existed long before the appearance of the Neanderthal man. The conclusions are that the Sapiens type has been there always. "For all these reasons it seems probable that neither Peking nor Neanderthal man represents the outcome of a process of human evolution."

There apparently existed alongside of each other Homo types as well as Homo Sapiens, but the latter because of his power of consciousness did not descend from less capable and intelligent ancestors. In my experience of mankind I have never come across two feebleminded parents who have produced children of higher intelligence. Lissner states : "When a museum displays models of Peking man, Neanderthal man and modern Homo Sapiens side by side, it encourages a conception of physical and intellectual development which is not in accord with the views of contemporary science."

This picture then sees Homo Sapiens as making his way down the millions of years, while parallel lines of lower strata of life accompanied him. Whether Homo Sapiens could have produced offspring by mating with Neanderthal is not known. But if fertilization took place from such unions, some lower species of the Homo Sapiens group might well have emerged. In the end the lower species and the Neanderthal became extinct while Homo Sapiens the carrier of a higher self consciousness continued his journey down the ages, perhaps because of the need for the evolution of this Sapiens consciousness.

In view of the inadequate conjectures of such eminent thinkers as Julian Huxley and the limitations he and others placed on their perspectives of life by confining these exclusively to the biological sphere those of us who take cognizance of the psi phenomena of man, and especially of his inner astral personality, and its ability to separate from the physical, are therefore entitled also to speculate about the origin of life on our planet. We have a richer world for our conclusions.

When we read of the people who have experienced psychic phenomena, and who have had to co-operate with non physical intelligences to obtain their results as in the case of the late Dr. Glen Hamilton, then we are driven to the realization that we are not the owners of life, but that we are possessed by it. In fact our wisdom depends on our adjustment to this ownership of life, and so we seek the meaning of things, and perhaps in consequence develop that disinterested curiosity which is science in our times.

The existence of the astral or inner personality and its manifestations to those capable of these extrasensory perceptions, as well as that degree of self consciousness which made the astral personality aware of its separate existence from the physical body and brain, made me seek for explanations other than the biological approach to life's manifestations.

Most people have the feeling or at most dim awareness that every person possesses an intuitive basis for his thoughts. Even those thoughts which come from facts of an objective nature are often coloured by some subjective intuitive interpretation of the mind, as if a little more light is added to the senses. The idea that somehow there existed an inner world of man beyond the physical appearance, slumbered in my mind from the early days with Outa Jantjes. Although he wove many fantastic tales for my amusement, there were some whose basic possibilities are widely accepted today.

Hence when it came to the time when I had to study comparative anatomy, and embryology I found these sciences could so easily be interpreted and explained by the Darwinian theory of evolution. But in spite of this smoothness of the superficial flow of scientific thought and its plausible correspondence, I strangely enough could not free my mind from the idea that the whole thing was an artefact. I had no prejudice against the theory only something inside me stood aloof from complete acceptance. There was always this question : where does the spiritual and full intellectual link with man come in? And even when one ingenious friend suggested that a thousand souls of small reptiles made the soul of an ape, and that a thousand souls of apes made the soul of Homo Sapiens, the fact remained that soul, mind and all these abstract qualities could only have been primary and not the products of matter.

I spoke to one of my professors about these doubts in my mind when we were alone one afternoon. He was impressed but advised me to become philosophical after I had passed my examinations and treat the theory of evolution as a means to an end. This was good Scottish wisdom. He admitted candidly that he had on spiritual grounds found an incompatibility the same as Wallace did.

In the course of time these vague intuitive mental aversions of my deeper mind found supporting evidence in psi phenomena, as well as in the writings of such thinkers as Ivar Lissner. The facts as they appeared to me contradicted the remotest possibility that life could be the product of inorganic matter.

It is assumed according to these scientific ideas on the subject, such as life coming from carbon atoms, that there was no purpose at the back of life. It came in a random manner and purely by chance, and then from inanimate material produced the organic, the mind, the consciousness and the soul. All of these were mere derivations from the original carbon atom. Such an idea could only make sense to anyone who had in the first instance excluded psychic life as a reality in its own right and secondly as the ultimate spiritual reality of man.

Man has existed on this planet for untold millioms of years, and if he has been Homo Sapiens from the beginning then he had his psychic equipment and capacities from that time. He would thus have had clairvoyance, telepathy, precognition, telekinesis and trance conditions with manifestations of ectoplasm, as well as mystic visions, and communications with those who had died. Indeed it is my firm belief that he has had all these functions and phenomena from the dawn of his existence.

And from that time the psychic sensitives in the group were the leaders of healing and religious life. One would therefore expect that man's basic curiosity in those days nearest his origin would have been concerned with his advent or origin on this planet. The whole picture of ancestral worship in ancient and archaic times came perhaps from memories recaptured by the psychic sensitives of those days.

These memories very likely formed the fundamental material of man's early religious aspirations and practices. He knew in the beginning about the reality of his psychic life, and the existence of other planes or dimensionalities for his life after his earthly existence. In all simplicity he considered that these future states were in the sky. But what is more is that in archaic times man believed that his ancestors came from the sun. Now since the sun is a star they therefore believed in the stellar origin of the first Homo Sapiens. His subsequent astrology was probably a by-product of assumption.

These solar ancestors of earth-man gave rise to the wide-spread belief among people and cultures in different parts of the world that they came from the sky, and that their rulers were children of the sun. Why should man conceive of such an idea, so exalted and abstract if his immediate ancestors were anthropoid or primate types? The answer is not difficult if we do not lose sight of the fact that from the earliest times man had his mediums, his prophets and soothsayers. Some of them could have received enlightened insight with regard to the origin of life.

To understand this amazing system of belief among the diversities of cultures in most ancient times, one should read that remarkable book "The Children of the Sun" by W. J. Perry, M.A. who was reader in cultural anthropology at the University of London. It contains research and clear thinking of the highest order. We find from his investigations that the adoration of the sun was spread almost all over the world, even to the tribes of North America and to the borders of Lake Superior.

When the Aryan speaking people invaded India they found that the rulers of the Asuras and Nagas claimed that they were descendents of the Children of the Sun. They were originally divine beings and incarnations, so they believed, of the Sun-God himself. These differed from the kings of the Aryans who merely believed that they had divine descent. But even in America the earliest kings were said to have descended from the sun as offspring of the Sun-God.

We have therefore historical evidence of this wide-spread archaic belief that at some time in the beginning the first people came from the sun. These children of the sun could fly through the air and visit other worlds in the sky. They were said to have been divine beings who were incarnated as men. Once they became more materialized they were considered semi-divine. Always there was the sky world to which they returned after death.

Then there were the archaic ideas about creation which conceived of all life as having been derived from the sky to which it would ultimately return. We know of course that Ra the Sun-God of Heliopolis was looked upon as the actual father of the king. We must also credit the Egyptian priestcraft with the ingenuity to use this origin to enhance the prestige of their kings as part of the religious adoration.

W. J. Perry mentions that "According to the Heliopolitan theory life was an emission of vitalizing light, and of a creating word. Ra the Sun-God was the creator par excellence. The two creative crafts, pottery making and the carving of statues have come to be associated in Egyptian thought with the idea of the creation of men." We find then in all these beliefs of the origin of man that he took on matter and that life in its fullest sense was lived after death in the sky.

When however we bear in mind that mediums or psychic sensitives played a dominant part in the shaping of man's thoughts, and beliefs about life as we observe in the Bible, then we can understand the prominent place in man's mind the underlying spirituality of man occupied in those days. For instance in the Rig Veda all life is held to come from the sky. Man's soul is his breath which at death returns to the sun.

Now our sun is just one star among myriads of stars, and each star must be regarded as a huge power-station which generates energy in its interior and pours this energy out into space in the form of radiation from its surface.

Our sun for instance has an output of fifty horsepower per square inch. Now since radiation has weight the sun pours out four million tons of radiative energy every second. And although I have no scientific basis for this intuitive assumption I believe the sun has an energy economy system, and that it cannot run down, but is capable of generating energy by a building-up process in its interior. A process which might be closely connected with death on this earth and on other planets which possess life.

Since science has speculated about the origin of life on this planet, and reached no explanation which we can accept because of the evidence in favour of the existence of an inner personality, I think I am entitled to advance a theory based on the beliefs of the children of the sun as to the origin of life here. My intuitive conception has woven itself around the existence of the astral personality.

The word astral means coming from the stars, and it has always puzzled me why this particular name was given to the projection of the inner personality from the physical body. Paracelsus for instance assumed that man had an astral body which explained the occurrence of presentiments. But the term has a definite stellar association, and I do not consider that this association is recent, say as far back as the time of Paracelsus. I think this idea of an inner personality capable of stellar existence or existence in an inner dimensionality of our sun is the original memory or knowledge of man's stellar origin.

Let us imagine that the astral plane is actually located in the sun, and that the energy system which is organized as the astral vehicle of the Ego is composed of a substance coming from the interior of the sun, but that this energy system permeates the whole universe in various densities or concentrations. When the astral properties of our sun millions of years after it came into being reached the stage for sustaining astral life forms, these astral beings were drawn by some sort of magnetic attraction from the next senior and nearest star in our galaxy.

Representative astral life forms from other suns in the milky way might also have been attracted so that the stars with astral frog life, spider life, bee or other insect life, vegetable life and even those with homonid or ape life types all made their contributions to our planet either directly to the planet or first to our sun as the source from which the next process would take place. Our sun could have been a Noah's Ark or a veritable cosmic museum of astral life forms.

After the formation of our earth and perhaps while still in a gaseous state a magnetic attraction took place which brought these astral forms into the atmosphere of the sun which probably included the earth's gaseous state of that time. Then as the cooling began the first astral genes of vegetable life began to assume ectoplasmic forms. The appropriate radiation from the sun which brought these astral life forms to our atmosphere could have been the vitalizing light which formed such an important part of the genesis of the Heliopolitan priests. From the genus of vegetation came the abundance of species of plant life changing gradually as conditions allowed from astral to ectoplasmic matter and then finally to the physical matter of our day.

The ectoplasmic forms could have attracted by electromagnetic means the interstellar atoms of a material nature which then became our most external form of matter. This process of becoming physical went through the stages of astral and then astral taking on ectoplasmic substance, and then ectoplasmic accumulating interstellar dust or atoms to become physical forms. This process could have taken eons of time.

One factor which is of great importance is the composition of our earth's atmosphere and the nature of the light which reached the earth from the sun. The protective gaseous layers containing ozone and the dominance of light of the ultraviolet and red varieties could very well have promoted the development of ectoplasmic forms as we have found in our seance rooms.

The rudimentary ectoplasmic life forms lived on the nourishment of the earth's atmosphere, and so breathing was probably the main channel for nurture. Perhaps herein lies the origin of the idea which associated the soul with breath, a memory which came from the period when astral ectoplasmic clad life forms or creatures lived entirely on the air of that time.

The vegetation prepared the way for insect and reptile and so came genus after genus in the process of materialization as if dropping from the sky in accordance with the suitability of conditions for survival in outer physical form. From the ectoplasmic stage probably came the material protoplasmic stage. The one prepared the way for the other until the Homo types and Homo Sapiens walked the earth.

At first then the gaseous content of the atmosphere and the nature of light was such that astral forms could take on ectoplasmic substance. Only when all forms were physically materialized did the change of atmosphere occur as part of the earth's evolution and the blend of different wavelengths of the constituents of light took place and became what it is today.

Looking at the beliefs of the archaic people and their origin from the sky and particularly the sun in this light one can see the reason why they credited their ancestors with flying through the air and visiting other places in the sky world. Only the knowledge that man has an astral personality which can be projected and which can exist by means of its own life independent of a physical form lends logic and reasonable thought to the ancient beliefs of the Children of the Sun.

At first one can picture a process where the astral forms would take on ectoplasmic substance by degrees and then dematerialize this form of matter according to gaseous and light conditions until ultimately the ectoplasmic form became a stable part of astral life in the earth's atmosphere or sky world. Then as the protoplasmic stage came to protect the ectoplasmic substance man no longer lived by breathing alone but sustained himself by ingesting the most ethereal contents of the fruits of vegetable life.

The impressive evidence of embryology when looked at with faith in the theory of evolution need in reality not be evidence of evolution in the Darwinian sense, but really a correspondence in accordance with the laws governing astral or stellar life. The explanation for similarities could mean that they shared the same life stream, but became differentiated according to genus, and the characteristic consciousness of each genus, and each individual including the self consciousness of man as a personality.

It is fascinating to imagine stars where the dominant life form is a spider or an ape. There could be planets belonging to stars in our milky way where these lower creatures on our earth are superior beings in their own worlds. But to come back to this amazing psychic life of man. Once these astral beings had materialized as physical beings their matings led to offspring, now where did the spiritual components of the Ego of the offspring come from?

There is of course the ancient association of man's soul with the breath and this has led to many forms of superstitious beliefs in degenerate peoples. Outa Jantjes for instance believed that the soul was drawn into the child when he took his first breath and many whites hold the same belief. If man came to this world in astral form and lived by breathing alone for ages, a probable inheritance of a racial memory or distortions of the original ideas could quite easily identify soul with breath.

The metaphorical conceptions of the ancient Egyptians presented the masses with the existence of a god Shu who was the god of breathing. In the "Egyptian Book of the Dead" Shu says: "I am Shu who conveys the breathing. I give air to the younglings as I open my mouth." If the people thought that the soul of the child was derived from Shu then it is a simple association of soul and breathing and this idea no doubt was shared by Outa Jantjes' race.

Among the primitive Arunta tribes of Australia they did not associate man's soul with generation by means of the sex act, but believed that the spirits of children were travelling in a whirlwind. Strangely enough I remember as a boy old coloured people describing a whirlwind as a wandering homeless spirit. But among the Arunta this belief had a powerful influence. It is said that when a native woman who did not wish to have a child saw a whirlwind approaching, she would flee for her life to avoid impregnation. Similarly these women were careful to avoid going through a gorge or ravine through which the wind came in a gush in case they should become impregnated.

Whatever these primitive superstitious relics of mind may be as derivations of archaic beliefs or knowledge, it is necessary for our modern scientific intelligence whether religious in an orthodox or unorthodox manner or not at all to examine this problem, and the evidence which claims a spiritual survival from the point of view of the association of a spiritual Ego with the natural process of procreation between man and woman.

To ask for the place of man's psyche in the sperm of man and the ovum of woman is to enter the crucible of mystery. Nevertheless man has a psychic nature, all we need to speculate about is how it grows from the union of male sperm and female egg cell. Let us picture what actually does take place during the mating of man and woman. The male introduces into the female reproductive organ from 300 to 500 million of male sperm cells. This extravagant and abundant projection of male sperm cells seems a complete and utter waste, because only one sperm cell is required to fertilize the egg and produce a child and only one does this. Hence why this wastage?

We have a picture of a profusion of sperm cells chasing one little egg cell and one would expect tremendous competition and yet out of these millions only one sperm cell and one only enters the female egg cell. The sperm is composed of a tiny nucleus, the rest is composed of a jelly-like substance called cytoplasm and probably identical with that which the first ectoplasmic forms acquired on earth. This jelly-like body ends in a little tail which enables the sperm to behave like a tiny snake and wriggle or swim along.

Now it is amazing to think that out of the 500 million sperms deposited one of these somehow streaks ahead, and when it meets the female egg usually in the tubes leading from the womb to the ovaries, it enters into an immediate and intimate union with the egg cell. In fact it buries its head deep in the egg cell and then its nucleus unites with the nucleus of the egg cell. Here without poetry or romance this blending of the two nuclei can be a union of two tiny souls guided by inner affinities.

We are immediately confronted with a situation for which to my mind biology has not provided an adequate explanation. The profusion of 500 million sperm cells of which one survives to fertilize the egg cell is not an act of blind extravagance. There is a law operative here whose mysterious nature we do not understand. In the first instance must we credit these cells with some incomprehensible nascent consciousness. Then to understand the success of one out of 500 million and the death of the rest we must assume that some power of attraction operated between one particular sperm and the particular female egg cell.

If for instance there are different electromagnetic charges in the sperm and the egg, that is if the egg is positively charged and the sperm negatively charged, then part of the success of the sperm is explained by the power of attraction radiated by the egg cell, but then this crude and generalized pull would be exercised on all 500 million and they would all plunge into the egg cell to fertilize it. Hence I consider that apart from the general law of the positively charged egg cell attracting the negatively charged male sperm cell there is another factor of tremendous importance.

While we roam in this domain of fact and speculation the outstanding impression remains that one particular sperm cell leaves his millions of competitors behind, as though they have given up the chase and are prepared to disintegrate for purposes not yet known. It could be that some chemical factor is absorbed from them into the female metabolism. But the choice by the ovum of one particular sperm cell could only mean one thing, and that is that the sperm cells all have different frequency rates of vibration in accordance with their spiritual genes. Hence the sperm cell whose vibration is identical with that of the ovum will overcome all the hazards to reach its goal.

It is not the health and vitality of the sperm cell or the egg cell which counts otherwise only the strongest and fittest of a species would be born. No, it is another law of affinity, a law of shared vibrations of the inner life of genes which makes man a mystery. Immediately this union takes place the nuclei of the cells, their little power-stations in fact, begin the process of creation. Now we know that each nucleus contains elongated bodies very much resembling strings of beads when viewed under a microscope.

These bodies are known as chromosomes and arranged along these chromosomes are invisible charges of dynamic energy and these are called genes. These invisible or shall we call them disembodied units of power constitute the essential power which determine the hereditary characteristics of the offspring. They reincarnate ancestral or parental characters and qualities in the offspring and subsequent generations.

These genes are the most mysterious units in the laws of procreation and the formation of personality. Their qualities and dynamics are such that they are passed from parent to offspring and as the offspring in turn becomes parent he passes them on to his children. By these means personal characteristics of a physical or mental nature could be reproduced in the offspring. In fact the personalities of ancestors are often seen in their subsequent generations.

I think that this law of the gene led to a great deal of confusion in ancient times, and was not at all understood by the archaic philosophical and so-called occult thinkers. These people must have been puzzled by the similarities with parents and remote ancestors which reappeared in the offspring and perhaps members of the second generation. It is highly probable that this repetition of ancestral characters and personality types led to the conclusion that the only valid explanation is the rebirth of an ancestral spirit in the body of a child. Such a conception could have formed the original basis for the idea of reincarnation.

Usually the gene is thought of as the carrier of this or that quality, such as temperament, endocrine gland endowment, emotional drives, blue eyes, colour of skin and a host of other factors belonging to the physical personality. But when we approach this mysterious gene with our knowledge of the astral personality, and also the ethereal atoms which the Ego will utilise in its evolution and progress in consciousness, then even these ectoplasmic, astral and more ethereal forms of energy substance must form part of the contents of the gene, and be transmitted to the offspring.

Once we accept the evidence which is not only abundant but also convincing that there is survival of personality in astral form after death, and we consider the affinities of vibrations between sperm and egg cells, as well as the reincarnation of physical and mental genetic qualities, then we should consider the possibility of the existence of spiritual family groups, or related spiritual groups coming from the same spiritual genetic stock.

Now if there are such spiritual family groups in whom the spiritual qualities are identical then the spiritual genes of a group in the germ plasm of man could give rise to similar drives and aspirations as well as talents in the physical personalities of people who have no earthly family relationship.

Again since energy is indestructible and since mass or matter and energy are the same then the substance whether physical, ectoplasmic or astral which formed the bodies of remote spiritual ancestors must still be in the universe and could thus be drawn or attracted to the spiritual nucleus of the Self and so form a vestment or body resembling the reincarnation of one who lived in ancient times.

When we apply the genetic laws of heredity to all the other higher forms of organized energy in the spectrum of life, and we include spiritual genes as well, then reincarnation does not become rebirth of a spirit in another body, but a question of inheriting identical spiritual and mental qualities of remote ancestors. One could picture the spiritual genetic group as a tree with buds and flowers along its branches. The old flowers die and the new buds blossom but they all resemble each other.

So the main spiritual and mental characteristics and talents of an ancestor could be regrouped around a new Ego, and virtually reproduce the personality of ages ago. The genes might even contribute to some sort of racial memory carried perhaps in the astral genetic units. Whatever the hidden truths of our beings we cannot help but stand in wonder when we reflect on the process of reproduction from the first moment that the life impulse brought the sperm and ovum together, and so within the germplasm of man packed the invisible, incomprehensible and intangible organizations of energy which made social man.

This Ego which comes into being when the nuclei of the sperm cell and the ovum merge becomes the main channel by means of which life organizes and expresses consciousness. The question is what sort of consciousness would the child have while carried in the womb? After all the usual earthly sensory consciousness could not possibly function. The child is not receiving sense impressions of sight, hearing, touch and taste from the outside world.

If sensations are registered they could only be those of warmth and comfort. Now if such a child should die before birth or at birth what is the nature of the consciousness that would survive, or would it disintegrate into separate energy units or systems? Or would this germinal or nascent inner consciousness of the child in the womb be of an entirely different order than that awareness which grows out of the senses and experience by means of the brain. Could this non sensory consciousness be entirely astral and therefore include the idea of a Self or I?

If the individual can survive with an astral consciousness without ever having lived outside the womb to obtain experience via his senses, then growth and development of the Self must take place on the astral plane and in the astral form. The following experience rather suggests that individual development of consciousness and intelligence does take place on the astral plane.

On a visit to London before the last war I decided to arrange a sitting through the good offices of the "British Spiritualist Alliance" with the medium Miss Lily Thomas. I obtained her name from a colleague who had had rather a remarkable sitting with this medium. I stipulated that I should remain anonymous and had to wait a few days as Miss Thomas had to come to London from the country. On the afternoon of my appointment I awaited her in a large high-walled room of an old English house having large windows draped with dark-red curtains I think.

Miss Lily Thomas entered the room while I was sitting in a deep armchair. She had a most pleasant and charming personality with that fresh complexion of the English country dweller. Her kindly eyes and pleasing smile created a sort of sparkling mental atmosphere. There was indeed something psychically immaculate and really trustworthy about her. She was not the sort of person who could be suspected of being artful because there was such a simplicity of innocence in the impression which she unconsciously made on me.

She informed me that it was her custom to say a little prayer before her sittings. I raised no objection and merely nodded. She bowed her head and her lips moved slightly. I heard no words. When she raised her eyes they were focussed almost beyond me. They seemed to stand still, caught up in some suspended distant gaze in the midst of nearness. She began speaking in a pleasant voice about a message from a deceased brother of mine.

At this a feeling of annoyance crossed my mind. I thought that she was deceiving me and was guessing and fabricating because I had no knowledge of a deceased brother, and in a family such as mine was it would have been quite impossible for me not to have known about such an event. I thought well I had met with fraud, as I was convinced that no member of my family had died at that time. Whether Miss Thomas sensed my feelings of antipathy I did not know but almost immediately she said that this deceased brother was fully aware that I did not know about his death.

He went on to say that he had been stillborn two years before my birth. He attributed his death to strangulation by means of the umbilical cord, as the doctor only arrived on the scene hours after the delivery had been attended to by a midwife. He reminded me that in those days the doctor had to travel sandy roads by means of a Cape cart drawn by six horses.

The latter was not news to me although they were impressive coming from the lips of Miss Lily Thomas. Nevertheless I could not accept the information that my mother had had a stillborn son before me. I had never heard a word about it and I felt sure that my mother would have told me about such an event. I was always under the impression that we were three sisters and three brothers. I decided however to deny nothing and to wait and see what else my supposed stillborn brother had to say. I did not believe the story.

But again, as if he or Miss Thomas were aware of my inner thoughts he said that I must enquire of my mother upon my return to South Africa and she will corroborate his birth and manner of death. I agreed more to encourage him than in faith in the possible truth. It seemed to me quite impossible that no one in our family had ever mentioned such an event.

He went on to describe how he grew up in the next world and how he and I were not only physical but also spiritual brothers. In fact we were so alike that if he had lived we would have appeared as identical twins. He shared my abstract and philosophical interests, and was often a source of my inspirations and intuitive conceptions. His development on the other side was primarily one of consciousness. Then towards the end of his communication he said : "Don't forget to ask your mother what she prayed for after my birth," and with that the sitting came to an end. I left and have never set eyes on Miss Lily Thomas again.

Strangely enough although I saw my mother several times a year in spite of her living five hundred miles away, I attached so little importance to this communication that I never mentioned it to her or forgot to inquire from her whether she had ever had a stillborn son two years before my birth. Then came an evening in 1943. I was writing to my mother and as she had not been well, I wrote her a long chatty letter about my children and their doings. While thus occupied I suddenly felt intruding on my mind a picture of the room in which I had had a sitting with Miss Thomas.

I could recall all the details, even the appearance of Miss Thomas and then the communication of the supposed stillborn brother. I experienced a strong urge to write and tell my mother all about it, and to ask her if the story were true, and what she had prayed for after his death. Well what was my surprise when a week later I received a letter from her corroborating in every detail the manner of his death. Mother thought I knew about it, but she could not remember ever having told me. With regard to the question about her prayer, she remembered being somewhat depressed after she lost this child, and that she prayed that she might have another son who could fulfill in this life what the stillborn one would have done if he had lived. Two years later I was born. She added that although she did not overtly express a belief in such communications as I had received from Miss Thomas, she felt that what Miss Thomas had told me could not be anything but the truth.

We subsequently discussed this communication alleged to have come from a child who was evidently dead when he was born. We in particular talked about the impressive facts of this case, which I felt had to be faced and traced to their logical conclusions.

In the first case there was a stillborn brother. Secondly my mother prayed for another son. Thirdly I had no conscious knowledge of the stillborn brother, nor of my mother's particular motive for the prayer. Fourthly I had never met Miss Lily Thomas before, and she knew nothing about my family in South Africa. It would be easy to say that she obtained this information by means of telepathy, but I candidly doubt such elaborate telepathy including the mentioning of a special prayer, when I who was in close proximity to Miss Thomas knew nothing about these facts.

It might be said that in some undefined telepathic manner Miss

Thomas established contact with my mother's mind, but without any object for psychometric vibrations, and without any knowledge of my mother we must dismiss such speculations. It could of course be that Miss Thomas obtained her information from a Universal Mind or some astral memory plane of our earth but then these records of the astral memory plane were corroborated by my mother, and if they were true for certain facts they should equally be true for the survival of an entity who claimed he was stillborn.

If on the other hand Miss Thomas gained access to a Universal Mind and received the information from such a source, then again the authenticity cannot be denied, for what reason would a Universal Mind have for communicating an untruth about survival of my discarnate brother and tell the truth about all the other events connected with his birth, including my mother's desire and her prayers. Logic in this instance stands four-square behind the fact that such an event occurred, and that the evidence in favour of his survival of death is overwhelming.

This evidence about this stillborn child leads one to conclude that there is a continued existence of the fundamental human Ego. The astral body and the ectoplasmic formations and materializations including those mentioned in the Bible hence give substance to the conception that the Ego acquires different bodies or vehicles of expression according to the energy organization of the plane or heaven in which it has its existence.

One day science might acquire sufficient data about life to include these concepts in the study of psychobiology. Taking this communication of my stillborn brother as an authentic example, then one has to conclude that his spiritual maturity and growth of consciousness occurred on other worlds, planes or heavens of existence. In short that the development of his Ego's consciousness took place on abstract planes. This evolution then implies a progressive growth of a wider comprehension and inner view of the energy systems of the universe. This is perhaps one of the necessities why science should embrace a psychobiology of discarnate life and existence.

When one judges by the supernormal psychic experience of people then it does appear that there is a law which determines the plane which is appropriate for the particular consciousness at the time of death—in fact a strong suggestion of a state of resonance or intunement between the mind of the deceased and the ethereal state or density of the plane which will receive him. St. Paul for instance in his descriptions of his mystic and clairvoyant experiences also provides evidence of abstract planes of existence. But I cannot recall once having heard a Christian sermon where these Biblical statements were expounded as stages of discarnate evolution.

For example in the second epistle of Paul to the Corinthians Chapter 12 verses 1 to 6 he speaks as follows :

1. "It is not expedient for me doubtless to glory. I will come to visions and revelations of the Lord."

2. "I knew a man in Christ above fourteen years ago, (whether in the body, I cannot tell; or whether out of the body, I cannot tell : God knoweth;) such an one caught up to the third heaven."

3. "And I knew such a man, (whether in the body, or out of the body, I cannot tell : God knoweth)."

4. "How that he was caught up into paradise, and heard unspeakable words, which it is not lawful for a man to utter."

5. "Of such an one will I glory : yet I myself I will not glory, but in mine infirmities."

6. "For though I would desire to glory, I shall not be a fool; for I will say the truth : but now I forbear, lest any man should think of me above that which he seeth me to be, or that he heareth of me."

Verse six makes it clear that St. Paul was speaking of his own personal experience. There is great emphasis on the words "Whether in the body or out of the body." With the knowledge of astral projection, clairvoyant perception, or mystic experience as excursions of consciousness at our disposal, we are in a position to interpret and analyse St. Paul's amazing statement, and draw certain valid conclusions based on Biblical authority.

He tried to convey the idea that there was a difference between his physical self and his inner Ego or Self. He states : "But now I forbear lest any man should think of me above what he seeth." He therefore had experienced a clearer consciousness in his inner or astral self, and he did not want to confuse his audience by making them credit his physical self with what he performed in his astral personality and its more profound perceptions. He lays stress on the point that he was not quite sure whether he was in his body or out of his body. It meant therefore that the reality of being out of one's body was accepted by him. He knew the truth of such an existence otherwise he would not have mentioned this possibility for visiting other planes of life.

It could of course have been a clairvoyant experience or a mystic vision, but the words "caught up to the third heaven" do not mean a revelation of the third heaven, but must be read to signify that his inner or astral self was projected and drawn into that plane. A great deal more however can be read into these words of St. Paul, not only did he maintain that the glory of this experience belonged to his inner, and not his physical self, but by his statement he affirmed that he knew of other planes of existence for discarnate life.

He declared it as the truth that he visited the third heaven, which could be interpreted as meaning the third from the earth plane. If then he visited a third heaven, as a name for a non-physical plane then his statement implies a first, a second and a fourth and so on. Hence St. Paul verifies the conception of a hierarchy of planes of non-physical progress and evolution for discarnate man.

Here then we have an authoritative Biblical statement by a psychic sensitive such as St. Paul was, that there are other planes for the manifestation of life. In fact when we read the work of the pioneers in psychic research life those of Professor Richet, Dr. Osty, Sir William Crookes, Dr. Baron von Schrenck-Notzing, Dr. Geley, Dr. Glen Hamilton, Sir Oliver Lodge and a host of other famous people trained in the principles of science, and we include the experiences of astral projection, and especially those of Sylvan Muldoon, we find to our pleasant surprise many of their equivalents mentioned in the Bible.

The spiritistic hypothesis which Dr. Glen Hamilton and other research workers found indispensable for obtaining results of a certain nature, therefore implies co-operation of minds across the barriers or energy systems insulating one world or heaven from another, and from our earth's sensory intellectual consciousness.

When we read accounts of psychic phenomena and psychic experience in the Bible, and we listen to the mention of them by the leaders of the various creeds, we are left with the impression that these things only happened at that time, and in that era because of the glory and holiness of the beings with whom they were associated.

In fact the impression is conveyed that they are dated and cannot recur again. They belonged to a time of miraculous powers and manifestations completely supernatural. But some of us know that these impressions are wrong. In fact these false impressions should be corrected because the psychic phenomena of Biblical accounts have occurred in modern times, and in laboratories of men whose one quest was the search after the truth.

Our conception of a hierarchy of life or what I have called a spectrum of life's energy systems, therefore consists of heavens or planes for the discarnate, and as stages for the continuous development of the consciousness of the Ego. The experience which St. Paul had was so overwhelming and so ethereal in its significance that he thought it quite beyond the comprehension of his hearers. So he said "and heard unspeakable words, which it is not lawful for a man to utter." We have then no means of picturing these further heavens of the hierarchy of life, except occasional mystic flashes of insight and a dim intuitive awareness of these higher refinements of thoughts and feelings.

Nevertheless, a little reflection will show that the deeper inner views of one's Ego do possess qualities which belong to a higher life, for in spite of the many factors which can retard and arrest its progress both here and in the denser astral regions, man's feelings of wonder, awe and reverence, as well as his aesthetic appreciations and his desire to use thought creatively all appear to be rudimentary steps towards a fuller life.

St. Paul made charity of heart one of the most essential mental qualities for a higher state of consciousness. I have often wondered whether he came to these conclusions as a result of his "unspeakable" psychic experiences and mystic visions? Because he said in 1 Corinthians 13 verse 2 : "And though I have the gift of prophecy, and understand all mysteries, and all knowledge; and though I have all faith, so that I could remove mountains, and have no charity, I am nothing."

It could mean that one's spiritual progress, that is the dynamic force for discarnate evolution on the astral plane requires the feeling-tones of natural kindness, goodwill and benevolence. To him these qualities when sincerely felt and cultivated are vital to ethereal life. It makes one wonder whether these are also the qualities which are necessary to prevent an earthbound state on the lower astral? It seems as though the growth of man's consciousness hereafter requires the dynamic qualities of this form of charity, as exemplified by the Red Cross.

Could a person really live with someone, choose him as a friend or companion if he is devoid of even the rudiments of charity of heart? Without these feeling-states the consciousness of one who has passed through death would probably be arrested and would remain preoccupied with its sensual and material values. It is difficult to imagine a person with a true aesthetic temperament who does not at the same time possess some trait of natural kindness. Perhaps St. Paul has laid emphasis on one outstanding mental quality which would assist in life's progress hereafter. There are others as well.

If on the other hand these charitable feelings of man rank on the same level as wonder, reverence and awe, then these higher qualities of man's psyche could be suppressed or overlaid by aggressive, destructive and other purely selfish motives, which in consequence arrest the influence of the charitable feelings or faculties of the Ego. Man's sojourn on the lower dense astral regions could therefore be brought about by such underdevelopment of these higher psychic functions, because our educational systems are unaware of their ultimate spiritual values.

When however the laws of monotony had caused a faint awakening of a desire for change then these higher faculties or functions of feeling begin to germinate, and as a result would give rise to a desire or wish to become part of a greater whole by means of sharing aesthetic values, love and sympathy. Qualities of this nature would be quite incompatible with any earthbound state or a sojourn in the lower regions of the astral plane.

When we consider these states of psychic arrest or retardation of the spiritual valuation of consciousness, we have I think to bear in mind the role of ectoplasm as a substance of life and a form of energy, which I consider intermediate between the astral and the gross physical energy system.

Normally therefore this ectoplasmic energy would be in close attraction to the astral body and would cling to it until its natural dissolution or disintegration occurs as an organized energy system. This dissolution I suppose should normally occur after death when the ectoplasmic constitute the energy of the astral cable or silver cord, and then becomes so attenuated as life departs that it snaps or separates completely, losing all magnetic hold on the protoplasm of the cells of the corpse.

But let us assume that the consciousness of the dying person is such that the qualities necessary for recognising the transition are absent and furthermore that the germinal qualities of charity on which St. Paul laid such stress are equally undeveloped, and that there are no memories or ideas in the astral mind anticipating a future life, or no abstract thought or feeling about such a possible discarnate existence, then one would expect such a being to be earthbound, and under such conditions it is highly probable that the ectoplasmic substance might adhere to the astral body. This would provide conditions for seeing ghosts or haunts in almost physical form, as a result of the density and law frequency of the adhesive ectoplasm.

There is evidence also which shows that astral beings of advanced degrees of consciousness could avail themselves of the ectoplasm of sitters in a trance, and so manipulate this energy to provide a tangible substance or cover for their astral forms. The appearance of Jesus to the doubting Thomas was a case in point, as was the materialization of little Rosalie.

These advanced discarnate beings know the art or science of concentrating, condensing and materialising ectoplasmic energy. And they are able to do so by means of techniques which have never been explained even to Dr. Glen Hamilton. He found however that the medium could not produce these phenomena by herself, but required this skill or science known to some discarnate beings. It could thus be that a great deal of the substantiality of the lower astral regions could be the result of concentrations of this ectoplasmic waveband of energy.

Man is accustomed to employ his sensory intellectual consciousness for the formation of pictures. It is necessary therefore to present one's intuitive imagination of the astral in some pictorial manner. The astral heaven or plane could thus be thought of as consisting after the pattern of the hierarchy of different regions of gradual diminution of density progressing towards ethereal planes of higher frequencies of vibration.

The evolution of the discarnate Ego and its consciousness who possessed charity of heart on earth in company with a religious nature would thus automatically seek the harmonious vibrations so as to resonate with the thoughts and sympathies of the discarnate entities of those heavens. It seems that the quality of sympathy has a refined effect on the human mind, and so makes us sensitive to feelings of a more reverential kind. Desire for discarnate sympathy hence promotes spiritual group life and evolves away from the carnal qualities of the lower astral regions.

But even the discarnate inhabitants of these earthbound and dense astral regions are subject to laws of change. They are merely retarded or undeveloped forms of consciousness. It seems logical to think that the monotony of repetitive existence must ultimately exhaust its energy. Even these beings would become bored with feelings of frustration, and one would think that at such a psychological moment the slumbering potentialities for advancement and change would awaken.

There is no reason why discarnate beings of advanced consciousness could not enter these lower strata of the astral to teach and enlighten these awakening minds how best to employ thought in that life. The Bible mentions that Jesus went to preach, I would say teach, the spirits who were in prison. Now spirits are not detained in earthly prisons, therefore this language clearly refers to those in earthbound conditions.

To understand this dynamic revealing nature of life one can imagine that the major task of the evolution of consciousness is the realization that the thinking principle of man must employ creative thought. This particular function of psychic life would really only truly begin as an exclusive development on the astral plane. Also this creativeness by means of thought working with the pliable astral energy must bring about an intense joy of self consciousness. The discarnate intelligence is at liberty to experiment with thoughtforms, while living with and within a cosmisc life substance.

Our earthly creative and constructive instincts are apparently drives, which come into a degree of fuller realization in these kindergartens of the higher astral regions. One could very well ask whether real abstract art in contrast to pictorial, photographic or representation of nature is not perhaps a reflection of astral interpretations of music, sound, force and energy organization. Maybe there too the aesthetic sense experiments with the decorative for the sheer joy of self-expression.

It is fascinating to think that a process of learning, adaptation and intunement with one's environment are dynamic forces, which pass over from earth-life with the Ego and evolve into higher forms of life. The Ego as a centre of consciousness, becomes as it were a power-house generating ideas which take form, shape and substantiality on the astral canvas. One can picture the sharing of pleasant feelings as astral beings delight in each other's creations in the processes of modelling with life.

In the face of this perspective of spiritual hope as an innate drive in the nucleus of one's Ego, stands the conclusions of physical science that ultimately we shall have the heat death of our universe. All its energy would be dissipated over billions of years hence. I suppose that suns or stars and planets, as organs of some Infinite Organism would be liable to the laws of change and disintegration.

But if life, and discarnate life at that, is a form of energy in circulation, then the external changes in the stars could very well be concerned with the interior evolution of discarnate life, and so the law of conservation of energy could have its spiritual counterpart. Who knows but that science has merely perceived one aspect of cosmic metabolism and has not yet discovered the counteragency of a building-up process. Cosmic radiation for instance does not come from the stars, but from the far-flung regions outside our stellar universe. Why should it not be part of a building-up process somewhere in the depth of the unknown?

If the astral system of energy is primarily generated by the interior of the stars and from there radiated throughout the universe, interpenetrating all space and all objects in space, and serving as the waveband for our extrasensory perceptions, then we can imagine a finite but unbounded universe with an energy economy of its own transforming physical man into higher psychical forms of intelligence. Viewing life from this perspective it could be probable that death on earth adds its quota of energy organized in discarnate form to the inner worlds of the stars, and so there is change but no death.

These ideas should not be considered as either impossible or improbable, because we need ideas, and it is only when we have an idea or an hypothesis that we have something from where to begin our creative thought or insight by means of the inner mind. Even science of the most objective kind cannot do without guessing or anticipation. Knowledge of truths already known by means of psychic research becomes the principal condition for the discovery of new ideas and truths. Science has always had the ability to set us free from the confines of the actual, and so has enabled us to penetrate beyond the regions of the possible. Our ideals are our mile-posts on this eternal course of life.

When I consider the astral life as the next stage on this journey, and credit it with the faculties that are here known as extrasensory perception, then I do so because of the known limitations imposed on mind by the brain of man. It is an amazing fact that out of the whole range of radiations known to science, and capable of being recorded by man-made instruments, only one part in ten thousand million is perceptible by the sensory organs of man. Scientific facts of this kind illustrate most emphatically that man's sensory intellectual consciousness provides him with only an infinitesimal fraction of the information available about the whole.

Is there any wonder then that man's mind is riddled with superstitions and ignorance about that vast field of life reserved for the power, the thought and the existence of the soul of man? One is reminded of the words of Robert Ingersoll : "Every cradle asks us 'Whence?' and every coffin 'Whither?'. The poor barbarian weeping above his dead, can answer these questions as intelligently as the robed priest of the most authentic creed."

Surely it is not meant that man's intelligence should only explore the physical planes of our worlds, and that his inner life, the source of his consciousness, and the purpose of the organization of his mind, and his ultimate psychic reality, should not fall within the honest scientific enquiries of man? The answer must be no, because it is only with the sensory intellectual consciousness that we can say with Whittier in his poem *Interlude After the Grave by the Lake* :

The life to be
Is still unguessed mystery
Unscaled, unpierced the cloudy walls remain
We beat, with dream and wish the
Soundless doors in vain.

Our age has produced undreamt of scientific achievements, and all are the products of man's thought and mind. But what emotions, feelings, ideas and motives are in control of the nuclear power that science has harnessed? Surely not those that our ideals have envisaged, indeed not the higher humanity for which Red Cross came into being, and for which the world produced a superior soul such as Henri Durant? *No*, it is a regressive mental control of the powers of nature. It is some immaturity of consciousness, dominated by a paranoid illness of some nations constituting the world mind.

Man has gone into space and in orbit around our earth. He aims to visit the moon, and has already sent rockets loaded with instruments into the depths of our solar system. Is he doing all this because space has become a scientific playground where each achievement enhances the paranoidal ego of a cold war wager? Or has he a drive for power which is becoming psychologically aberrant, because he has reached a phase in material progress and knowledge where the mind is in need of a higher inhibition in the hierarchy of consciousness?

In the absence of this superior directive of the spectrum of life in the mind of man, his destructive and aggressive impulses can only be controlled by an equal and opposite force. The terror of self-destruction by the forces of retaliation has kept the hand from pressing the button of nuclear war. Man has in a short space of time passed through two devastating, cruel and horrible wars, wherein all the vileness and crudities of impulse and thought could find expression and with what consequences? The barrel of the weapon has hardly cooled, and the genetic distortions of Hiroshima are not yet known, and yet man oblivious of past experience stands like an infuriated juvenile delinquent minus foresight and judgment, ready to hurl the next nuclear bomb.

What if this space race and this day and night competition in the production of greater and greater weapons for the total annihilation of man goes on and on? What will stop it? Surely not a change of mind and heart in those who know they possess power? Besides, what sort of change could one expect except some temporary change of front based on expediency for a breathing spell.

This then is the attitude the mind of man has reached by means of materialistic scientific culture. It is an inbalanced worldly psychological structure, and I believe it is inbalanced, because we have enslaved the thought of man in the shackles of material science and because the latter has become the nursery of the philosophers of our era. Therefore we can expect security and peace only as long as there is the stalemate of terror. We cannot expect peace from the noble aims of Red Cross until man has a consciousness which Red Cross can continuously cultivate for the maintenance of peace.

There is nothing to stem this onward rush of scientific discoveries, which all could be placed at the disposal of militarism. What if nations increase this reign of uncertainty and terror by placing nuclear weapons in orbit circling round and round our world, ready to be brought down over any city and destroy all its life by means of a mere radio signal. Must we continue to live in a world where paranoidism is on the rampage, and where civilized man's best brains are daily employed for self-defence. But I say we have a self-defence, and we can have the world's only effective weapon for that self-defence, and that is the cultivation of the right consciousness for Red Cross.

An analysis of the civilized global mind reveals nothing else than a state of mental confusion. We behold numerous creeds whose devotees seek the golden grail in the letter, because the pathway to the spirit is overgrown with fossilised thought. There is no intelligent question of Whence? and of Whither? And least of all is there any public need, any public awareness of a necessity to know what we are? If man himself cannot and has no desire to know in terms of clear logical knowledge what constitutes his being, and if the educated man does not demand this knowledge what can we expect from our seats of learning?

In consequence of this inarticulate mental state of man, this inability to ask What am I? we have been burdened with all sorts of strange cults providing answers for man's unconscious spiritual need for truth and knowledge, and often indeed very frequently these pseudo-scientific cults and organizations draw their followers from the lunatic fringe of society. Hence the supernormal is constantly finding supporters and bed-fellows who do not give respect and status to the position it ought to occupy in a world where man claims he seeks knowledge by honest disinterested curiosity.

University education should by now recognize as a universal necessity that a new dynamic of consciousness is required. Education should accept that the desire to know the significance of psychic phenomena is a valid need of man's intelligence. For inherent in such knowledge are the materials for a change in man's manner of thought and the feelings that should buttress his ethical values.

The mental instability of our world is evidence that we have neglected to probe deeper into the nature of man, because we have failed so far to discover the higher levels of the psychic hierarchy, which should inhibit and rechannel man's aggressive and destructive impulse life. We have long known that no religion, no creed or cult holds all knowledge. They might in some vague manner clothed in an abundance of verbiage and metaphor show the way to the truth but they do not provide stepping-stones of knowledge issuing from an honoured seat of learning and so helping man to realize there is a next plane of existence.

We therefore require a new science of psychobiology dealing with every aspect of psychic or psi phenomena, so that above all, the ectoplasmic part of life's spectrum can be studied, as well as the important role of the astral personality. It is incumbent upon all intelligent and educated people to realize that science is not bound to work only in a physical or material field. Science might become dogmatic, but it is never a dogma for it must always imagine, because its goals fall within the creative imagination. It is above all a product of man's thought.

We must hence use the power of thought and rescue science from its material incrustations, because as a creation of the thoughts of man we should demand a science which should have no plane of activity, no curiosity about life which excludes the discarnate forms and manifestations. In its strivings after the unknown it should have as a fundamental principle the conception that reality is not only the property of the objective and physical world.

The new psychobiology in pursuing the path of psychic research, will know how little ability we have to form ultimate values from commonsense impressions. It will also have to accept that the whole cosmos is an expression of energy in different wavebands of an infinite spectrum, and since this energy does become organized and is indestructible although capable of transformation, therefore man should know as a necessity whether intelligent conscious discarnate organized forms of energy can exist.

The peace of our planet demands that we equip man with a better consciousness for our ethical values—indeed a superior home for our ideals. This to my mind is the challenge of the inner man, and the subconscious higher humanity. For this purpose we require an enlarged science willing to investigate whether consciousness can exist independently of a physical organism? In its pursuits it can explore the outer space of the world and the inner space of the higher consciousnesss.

Such a larger and more comprehensive science of psychobiology will not be selfish as hitherto in only investigating its material subjects, but it will apply its knowledge that man presents a picture, which suggests that religion arises from an instinctive tendency in man to believe in, and to cultivate relations with superhuman agencies and powers, and secretly to desire to continue his life in some other form hereafter.

Such a conception would bring psychology clearly into the picture of psychobiological research, because of the fact that man has feelings of reverence, awe and wonder, which indicate an equipment for instinctively appreciating supernormal manifestations as inner potentialities of mind. In this manner psychobiological research will follow life and consciousness into their discarnate habitations, beyond our clouded perceptions, and beyond the insulating barriers of consciousness, which separate the brain man from the non-brain astral being.

This new psychobiology should follow life along its long unending trail into the regions of life's attenuation, where thought and feeling blend in their vibrations. Its quest will be to discover as much as possible about the truth of man. Such endeavours might become healing forces for man's mental life, and not only give us a clearer picture of spiritual man, but bring about a synthesis of knowledge embracing in its folds man's aspirations in the nature of mysticism, philosophy, psychology and religion.

In his three essays on parapsychology called *On the Edge Of Beyond*, Professor M. Valkhoff gives the following lines from Faust revealing the thoughts of Goethe :

Therefore myself to magic I give,
In hope through spirit voice and might,
Secrets now veiled to bring to light,
That I no more with aching brow,
Need speak of what I nothing know,
That I the force may recognise
That binds creation's inmost energies
Her vital powers, her embryo seeds survey,
And fling the trade in empty words away.

INDEX